Thrust Joint Manipulation Skills

FOR THE SPINE

Emilio J. Puentedura
PT, DPT, PhD

William H. O'Grady
PT, DPT, FAPTA

Forewords by
Laurie Hartman, DO, PhD
Joe Farrell, PT, DPT, FAPTA

Table of Contents

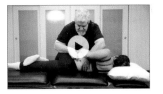

Video techniques found in Chapter 7 can be accessed at this web page:

OPTP.com/tjm-videos
Username: tjm
Password: techniques

The procedures and practices described in this book should be implemented in a manner consistent with professional standards set for the circumstances that apply in each situation. Every effort has been made to confirm accuracy of the information presented and to correctly relate generally accepted practices.

The author, editor and publisher cannot accept responsibility for errors or exclusions or for the outcome of the application of the material presented herein. There is no expressed or implied warranty of this book or information imparted by it.

Designed and published by OPTP.
3800 Annapolis Lane N #165
Minneapolis, MN 55447
800.367.7393 | OPTP.com

Copy edited by OPTP.

ISBN-978-1-942798-12-5

Foreword

Laurie Hartman, DO, PhD

I was very pleased when I was approached to write a foreword for a new spinal manipulation textbook to be authored by Emilio "Louie" Puentedura and William "Bill" O'Grady. I have been teaching manipulation for over 50 years, and met Bill 25 years ago at a course I was teaching in the United States. Since then, we have developed a great personal and professional relationship. He has attended several of my courses and we ultimately ended up teaching some courses together. I met Louie about seven years ago, through Bill at a course I put on in Las Vegas. He has also taught with me a few times. They both bring a unique and refreshing educational approach to manipulative therapy in their book. They bring their decades of experience and eclectic approach to provide students, experienced clinicians and educators with additional tools to enhance their abilities and provide effective, safe thrust joint manipulation.

Both of the authors have used their great combination of skill, knowledge, teaching and clinical experience in manual therapy to write this book. They have used many and varied methods applying their skills as clinicians to advance the knowledge and ability of the practitioner. Both are top-notch manipulators who have developed their own style of teaching, combining physiotherapy practice with osteopathic thinking. Both struck me as thoughtful and enthusiastic in embracing new concepts when I first met them.

It is apparent that a lot of thought has been placed in preparing this book. The chapters are written in a clear and concise fashion making it easier for the reader to absorb the information. The first chapter gives a great summary of the history of manipulation from ancient times to the present. The second chapter provides a thorough discussion on the evidence for using thrust joint manipulation (TJM). It provides an excellent bibliography including the most current published evidence.

The third chapter addresses the issues of safety in applying TJM techniques. This chapter provides a thorough background on both the safety concerns and research looking at each area of the spine. It gives a clear and concise view of the risks involved in manipulating the spine with the research to back it. Chapter 4 discusses clinical reasoning in applying TJM. The authors define clinical reasoning, the research behind it, its biomechanical and neurophysiological aspects and patient expectations. Finally, this chapter points out the importance of educating the patient in pain science as part of the treatment.

The next two chapters are unique to any book I have read on spinal manipulation. Chapter 5 has one of the most thorough set of drills that will prepare the clinician to safely and gently apply TJM. Some of the issues it addresses are the importance of amplitude, speed, palpation skills, use of the core, and effective use of large muscle groups in applying TJM. Chapter 6 provides the clinician with a description of individual tests recommended for each area of the spine that may help to rule out "red" and "yellow" flags prior to performing TJM.

Chapter 7, the techniques, is well organized and concise as well as unique. It gives a brief description of each technique, when to use it, which muscle groups to activate when applying each technique and recommended tests prior to performing the technique. The technique itself is divided into bulleted descriptions of patient and therapist position, contact points, position for the thrust and its application. Below each technique are clinical pearls, many of which I have used over the last 50+ years. This information is also provided in a concise manner, enabling the learner to fine tune their skills in order to effectively and safely apply each technique.

I know how much hard work has gone into producing the book and I know that you will learn and acquire as much knowledge and information from it as I did. The authors have written a book that is concise and easy to read. Their unique technique illustrations allow the learner to view both the patient and clinician positions from different angles. In learning a new skill, this book will go a long way. However, keep in mind that practice, practice, practice is the criteria to improve any skill; and with the use of this book, the practitioner is bound to be more successful with their treatment approach. I am pleased that Louie and Bill have used many of the principles and techniques that I have taught and incorporated them into their book. There are not a lot of new TJM books out there. I am delighted to recommend this book because of its unique approach, concepts and ideas. It should be part of every manual therapist's library.

Laurie Hartman, DO, PhD

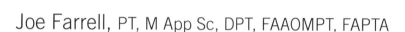

Joe Farrell, PT, M App Sc, DPT, FAAOMPT, FAPTA

As a founding fellow and first president of the American Academy of Orthopaedic Manual Physical Therapist (AAOMPT), practicing clinician for over 40 years, as well as a Senior Fellowship Faculty member of the Kaiser Northern California Orthopaedic Manual Physical Therapy Fellowship for nearly 35 years, I am very honored to write the foreword of this landmark book for Drs. Emilio "Louie" Puentedura and Bill O'Grady.

My connection to Bill dates to the early 1980s when he and I met through manual therapy colleagues in the Orthopaedic Section and our intimate ties to the Orthopaedic Specialty Certification (OSC) genesis, when I lead numerous item writer workshops for the OSC examination. Our professional relationship continued over the years with our involvement in the AAOMPT when Bill assumed the Chairmanship of the AAOMPT examination committee and in later years, Chair of the Orthopaedic Specialty Council. To this day, we engage in lively conversations relating to patient scenarios, teaching strategies and professional politics.

I first met Louie in the mid 1990s through our involvement in the AAOMPT. We bonded due to our Australian manual therapy training where I graduated with a post-graduate diploma in manipulative therapy (GDMT), Curtin University, Perth; and Louie from La Trobe University (GDMT), Melbourne. From afar, I have admired Louie for his prolific contributions to the research literature (over 60 peer-reviewed articles, two books and nine book chapters) and his teaching partnership with Bill over the past decade.

The authors have intertwined over the past 40 years of clinical experience and 30 years of teaching experiences within numerous levels of entry-level and post-graduate residency/fellowship education, and a professional and personal bond that has led to the creation of a "must-read" book on thrust joint manipulation for the spine.

The book is organized in concise, easy-to-read chapters with illustrated pictures and videos for quick reference to an array of useful thrust joint manipulation (TJM) techniques. Chapter objectives and outlines give the reader a framework for learning, and a "key point(s)" summary at the conclusion of each chapter also offers references/evidence for each chapter.

The first chapter offers a chronological history of manipulative therapy from ancient times to the present. The next chapter details a very up-to-date, evidence-based rationale including recent randomized clinical trials and systematic reviews for the everyday clinical use of TJM. Safety issues relating to use of TJM follow with, again, evidence-based rationale for the clinical utility of screening tests prior to TJM use.

A unique aspect of the book is an in-depth chapter on clinical reasoning as to when and why to use TJM, which is very often not reviewed, or for that matter, discussed in other orthopaedic manual physical therapy books I have read during my career. Another unique component is chapter five, which illustrates and discusses drills to develop thrust speed, effective stance and palpatory skills to assist clinicians of all levels of expertise with learning and teaching TJM. For all clinicians and teachers of manual therapy, the following chapter details the evidence-based routine tests and special tests which preclude the use of TJM at all levels of the spine.

The absolute gem of a chapter of this landmark book outlines the step-by-step of "how you should do it" for a multitude of TJM techniques. The authors offer, through their decades of clinical and teaching experience, a very concise description of the patient position, therapist position, contact points, position of thrust and application of the thrust. Additionally, they offer tips of how to fine tune the TJM technique and keys to successful performance of TJM techniques. The concluding chapter focuses on political issues revolving around TJM, legislative issues and the future direction of TJM education.

As a very experienced practicing clinician and fellowship senior faculty educator, I have had the privilege to observe some of the greats like Geoff Maitland, Freddy Kaltenborn, Stanley Paris, Laurie Hartman, Dick Erhard, Brian Edwards and Bob Elvey. I was mentored clinically by Edwards and Elvey and tutored in research by Dr. Lance Twomey, thus in my humble opinion, this book's credibility delivers to the reader more than I have ever read in a textbook about TJM. This book really matters if you are a student, clinician, teacher/educator or a researcher, due to the eclectic scholarly review of the evidence-based research relating to TJM, the clinical reasoning pertinent to TJM, and the step-by-step description of techniques which are not usually articulated in books of this nature.

In summary, my friends and colleagues, Bill and Louie, have delivered a landmark book on the skillful craft of thrust joint manipulation, a practice which has been clinically applied for centuries and continues to evolve as many clinicians and researchers around the world continue to prove its clinical value. This epic book will forever be on my office shelf and read and re-read for many years. It is a must-reference guide for any clinician or orthopaedic manual physical therapy educator.

Joe Farrell, PT, M App Sc, DPT, FAAOMPT, FAPTA
Danville, California 2017
Senior Fellowship Faculty
Northern California Kaiser Orthopaedic Manual Physical Therapy Fellowship

Preface

Emilio J. Puentedura, PT, DPT, PhD
William H. O'Grady, PT, DPT, FAPTA

When we sat down and discussed writing this text, our initial goal was to provide a user-friendly resource for physical therapy students and physical therapists wishing to learn how to enhance their thrust joint manipulation skills in the treatment of patients with musculoskeletal dysfunction in the spine. We have taught seminars and presented at physical therapy conferences on this topic for several years now, and over the past 10 years, we have also begun a line of research into the mechanisms, effectiveness and safety of thrust joint manipulation for the spine. We have wanted to share our knowledge and experience primarily within our own profession, and we certainly remain staunch advocates for thrust joint manipulation to the spine to remain within our professional scope of practice. However, our clinical and teaching experiences have shown us that best care of the patient with spinal pain and dysfunction should be the focal point for all manual therapy providers. Concerns about their safety and well-being told us that this information needed to be shared not only within our profession but also with all clinicians and personnel involved in providing thrust joint manipulation. Because of this, you will notice that we use the terms 'therapist' and 'clinician' throughout the text and not 'physical therapist'. Ultimately, we wanted to make thrust joint manipulation education accessible and relevant for all therapists to be able to safely and competently implement in their clinical practice.

There have been many great teachers of thrust joint manipulation techniques throughout the history of spinal manipulation. Although some physical therapists had been performing thrust joint manipulation since the birth of the profession more than 200 years ago, it has never been practiced by all physical therapists. Even today, it is not used in clinical practice by all physical therapists and, like many other areas of physical therapy such as pediatrics, cardiopulmonary, and neurologic rehabilitation, it attracts the interests of only a portion of the profession. Similarly, in other professions involved in the rehabilitation of musculoskeletal dysfunction, not all practitioners will regularly provide it as part of their clinical practice. This is probably because there are many other treatment interventions available to address spinal pain and dysfunction, but it may also be because of concerns about safety, skill and proficiency.

Thrust joint manipulation did not get widespread acceptance within the physical therapy profession in the United States until the 1960s and 1970s when clinicians like Stanley Paris, Dick Erhard, James Cyriax, Ola Grimsby, Freddy Kaltenborn, and others began teaching it. During that time, therapists were taught to introduce motion in the spine in three planes, using predominantly locking techniques to locate or engage the barriers for the manipulative thrust. These great teachers taught many great techniques, and it was amazing to the novice how well these master clinicians could move the spinal joints.

Both of us were novices in those times and it's interesting to think back to those days and realize there were unseen things they would do with their body and hands to augment what they were doing that they did not actually teach us. What were they feeling and how did they get such good control? They would demonstrate how to get from point A (start of the technique) to point G (the manipulative barrier) but they did not always show us points B, C, D, E and F, and how these points and what they were feeling at each point led them so accurately to point G. Unfortunately, there were a lot of steps in between points A and G that they did to perfect their technique, and they often did not explain or teach this to their students.

Dr. Laurie Hartman, DO, PhD, was one of the first teachers who discussed the subtleties of fine-tuning the manipulative technique using multiple vectors, stance, palpation, control, and the use of proper muscles and body mechanics to make the technique more effective and focused to a specific level. Although there is some (limited) research that suggests clinicians cannot be specific and focused to any specific spinal segmental level with thrust joint manipulation, we have seen plenty of clinical evidence to the contrary. Drawing upon our extensive experience and training in thrust joint manipulation, we will attempt to break down the components of an effective thrust technique so that you can learn how to provide safe, specific and focused thrust techniques. We will attempt to impart what you should be feeling and how your body and use of your core can affect the success of the technique. We will provide the best area of contact and other physical cues prior to applying the techniques with the goal of making the techniques most effective. Additionally, we will demonstrate more effective methods of palpation so that you will better understand what you are feeling.

Thrust Joint Manipulation Skills for the Spine contains chapters that will provide sufficient information about the components of a good thrust technique to allow all therapists engaged in the practice to understand and apply the concepts within the framework of movement-based therapy. The components of an effective thrust technique will include discussion of proper clinician stance and use of the core and proper muscles, speed, amplitude, palpation, patient position, direction, fluid body movement and control. This textbook will familiarize the reader with the concept of focusing to engage the barrier as it relates to patient comfort, and will provide clinical pearls along the way that should further enhance skill acquisition and technique.

In **Chapter 1**, we point out that thrust joint manipulation has been around for as long as mankind has suffered from joint pain and dysfunction, and how modern manual therapy has progressed to a more inclusive evidence-based framework. We stress that the colorful history of thrust joint manipulation may lead some healthcare professionals to believe it has no place in modern medical care. However, the fact that patients continue to seek this care and report improvement from it suggests we should not dismiss it entirely.

Chapter 2 provides a detailed discussion of the current scientific evidence for, and against, thrust joint manipulation to the spine. While there may be systematic reviews that suggest thrust joint manipulation is no more effective than any other intervention for spinal pain,

we contend that not all spinal pain and dysfunction is the same, and that some types respond rapidly and favorably to thrust joint manipulation. A critical appraisal of the evidence is provided so the reader can make more informed clinical decisions about which patient might respond best to thrust joint manipulation. Additionally, much if not all the research on thrust joint manipulation fails to truly provide it as the intervention of interest. "Manipulation," "spinal manipulative therapy," "mobilization" and "manual therapy" are often used interchangeably in many research designs. When thrust joint manipulation is examined as the intervention in any study, but it is not adequately described and its delivery not tightly controlled, it is no surprise that results are disappointing.

Safety with thrust joint manipulation is a significant concern for all therapists, and in **Chapter 3** we present a detailed discussion of the safety concerns. We include the two systematic reviews of case reports of adverse events following thrust joint manipulation to the cervical and thoracic spines that we authored, and present the case for sound clinical reasoning in the determination of appropriateness of using thrust joint manipulation techniques. We also discuss the results of a recent survey study of physical therapists in the US concerning their thoughts about thrust joint manipulation.

Chapter 4 provides detailed discussion of the clinical reasoning as to when and why we might use a thrust joint technique in the spine. We will cover the relevant clinical prediction rules, how they were developed and validated (if so), how they have caused some consternation and controversy amongst clinicians, and how they may be appropriately used within a clinical reasoning framework for best practice.

In **Chapter 5**, we provide some drills that will help develop speed, the proper use of the core, activating the proper muscles, effective stance and palpation skills. These are skills we have learned and practiced for more than 40 years and they are skills that many experienced clinicians have developed over time with repeated clinical practice. These are the drills we wish we had been taught all those years ago when we began learning thrust joint techniques, as we believe they enhance skill acquisition and lead to the development of expertise at a much faster rate.

Chapter 6 covers some of the physical tests that we consider to be an integral part of the patient examination. Prior to administering thrust joint manipulation, all clinicians should have completed a thorough clinical examination of their patient. It should include both a detailed subjective history of the patient's primary and secondary complaints, and a skilled physical examination of the patient's affected spinal region as well as related areas.

Chapter 7 is the 'how you should do it' section. It provides step-by-step descriptions of thrust joint techniques for the entire spine – from the atlanto-occipital joint to the coccyx. There are many techniques that we could have covered, but it is not the goal of this textbook to present every thrust technique out there. Instead, we have chosen those with which we have had the greatest clinical success. It is our belief that if you can learn a few good techniques for each spinal area, and perform them skillfully and safely, you will be better off than you would be if you used 50 different techniques that you could perform with only mediocre skill and success. With each technique, we provide a detailed description, and we note the primary muscles activated by the clinician during the delivery of the thrust. We provide some mechanical suggestions for when to use the technique and some special tests worth considering prior to using the technique. Each technique has clear descriptions of patient position, therapist position, contact points, position for the thrust, and application of the thrust. There are also photos and videos of each technique to provide visual aids to learning. Finally, we provide some notes on fine tuning and keys to successfully achieving joint cavitations for each technique.

To summarize, our goal with **Chapter 7** is to be able to break down the components of an effective thrust technique. To this end, the reader will be able to break down the parts of the technique enabling them to perform it both effectively and with the greatest comfort and safety for the patient. We provide helpful keys and clinical pearls with the goal of guiding the reader to a more successful outcome with each described thrust technique. Our goal is to instruct therapists on how to involve greater use of their body, as we believe this will allow the therapist to recruit larger proprioceptors that will aid in greater control in engaging the barrier.

Finally, in **Chapter 8**, we provide a conclusion, summary and some thoughts on the future direction of thrust joint manipulation education. We present a brief discussion on the politics and legislative efforts to limit the provision of thrust joint manipulation to specific practitioners, and why we believe those efforts will ultimately fail and why they *should* ultimately fail. Our central focus should always be what is in the best interest of the patients we care for, and as long as they are receiving benefit and moving on with their lives with less pain and disability, it shouldn't matter who used what to help them get there.

Neither of us knew much about thrust joint manipulation when we first graduated from physical therapy school. Each of us was introduced to it differently because of the time – Bill graduated in 1972 and I graduated in 1980 – and because of the location – Bill was in the USA and I was in Australia. However, both of us had our first exposure via a skilled osteopathic clinician, and it sparked our interest. From there, we soon found ourselves attending seminars and courses to acquire our novice skills in thrust techniques. Once we began using the techniques in the clinic, we soon had our share of successful outcomes but equally, we were left distressed by those patients who reported worsening of their complaints following our interventions. Learning about those unwanted side effects (luckily, neither of us ever caused any serious adverse events) following thrust joint techniques was an eye-opening experience. It forced us to reconsider the forces we were using with our thrust techniques, the amplitude of movement we were using, and other aspects that, over time, led us to experience greater success and almost no unwanted side effects or discomfort following our interventions.

We have thoroughly enjoyed using thrust joint techniques in our clinical practice and continue to enjoy teaching its finer points to clinicians at weekend seminars and conferences; and to our Doctor of Physical Therapy students at the University of Nevada Las Vegas. It is our hope that with this textbook, you will experience a similar sense of excitement for these techniques and how you might safely and effectively apply them in the appropriate patients.

Emilio J. Puentedura, PT, DPT, PhD, and
William H. O'Grady, PT, DPT, FAPTA

Chapter 1

History of Thrust Joint Manipulation

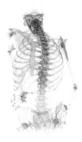

1.1: Chapter Objectives

The main point of this first chapter is to highlight the incredibly rich history of thrust joint manipulation (TJM), and to discuss how it has been practiced by mankind throughout the ages. The fact that it was continuously practiced throughout the ages should be a testament to its perceived clinical benefits. As the practice of medicine slowly modernized in the 1700s, TJM began to fall out of favor and its practitioners (the bonesetters) were viewed with skepticism and ridicule. But there is no doubt that patients receiving such treatment perceived some significant benefits that 'modern medicine' was failing to provide.

This set the scene for the founding of osteopathy and chiropractic in the late 1800s as new vehicles for the delivery of TJM within the slowly modernizing scientific and medical field. It should also be noted that early in the developing field of physical therapy, TJM was being provided to patients to restore joint motion and musculoskeletal health. The quest to more fully understand the clinical benefits of TJM led to the development of the various manual therapy approaches within the physical therapy profession. It is also important to appreciate the history and development of manipulation within the physical therapy profession.

1.2: In the Very Beginning

Imagine if we could travel back to the time of anatomically modern humans (*Homo sapiens sapiens*) some 50,000 to 25,000 years ago. We witness a pair of males returning to the family group after a hunt, carrying the fruits of their success slung on a pole across their shoulders. Imagine the possibility of this scenario playing out. As they journey back to their family group, one of the hunters complains to the other that carrying the fruits of their hunt all that distance has given him a pain in his back (Figure 1.2a). However, the other hunter doesn't offer any sympathy. He doesn't want to carry the animal carcass all that way on his own! Isn't it entirely possible that once back with the group, as they celebrate the success, another man in the group enthusiastically hugs the hunter with back pain from behind and lifts him up joyously? In the process, they both hear several audible 'pops' emanate from the hunter's spine, and immediately after this, his back pain is all but gone.

Could this have been the first, unrecorded episode of spinal manipulation in the history of mankind? It's not all that farfetched if you think about it. The point we are trying to make is that spinal manipulation is as old as mankind.

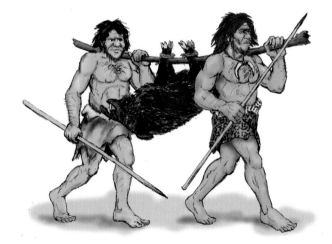

Figure 1.2a: According to anthropologists, *Homo erectus* and *Homo sapiens sapiens* may just be earlier and later varieties of the same species and therefore all should be called *Homo sapiens*.

1.3: Ancient Times

Walking on another individual's back for the relief of pain is a primitive method of manipulation that predates recorded history. However, the first recorded descriptions and illustrations of TJM are attributed to Hippocrates, the father of medicine (460-370 BC). In ancient writings, it is reported that Hippocrates used spinal extension (traction) and pressure (manipulation) on a back pain sufferer who was lying prone on a wooden table[1] (Figure 1.3a). Hippocrates is reported to have described spinal manipulation as 'rachiotherapy', saying it was an old art and that he thought highly of those who first discovered its importance and who would follow him in furthering the art of natural healing.[2] In his treatise on joints, Hippocrates spoke of *'parathremata'*, where 'the spinal vertebrae are not displaced by very much; only to a very small extent' and went on to say 'it is necessary to have a good knowledge of the spine, because many disorders are associated with the spine, and a knowledge of it is therefore necessary for healing a number of disorders'.[2]

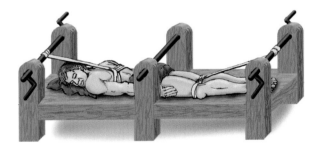

Figure 1.3a: The bench of Hippocrates, per Byzantine edition works of Galen in the second century, AD.

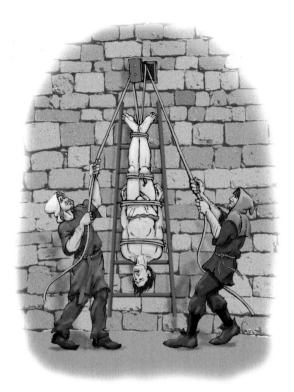

Figure 1.3b: Succussion was the practice of repeatedly shaking a patient, and in cases where patients were tied upside down, it was thought that traction might correct spinal misalignments.

It is also reported that spinal traction methods were practiced in the days of Hippocrates. Here, the patient would be tied upside down to a rack that was attached to ropes and pulleys along the side of a wall or building. These ropes were pulled to elevate the patient and then released, whereupon the rack would crash to the ground and the patient would receive a distractive thrust to their spine.[3] This was often done repeatedly and was termed "succussion" (Figure 1.3b).

Almost 600 years after Hippocrates, Claudius Galen (131-202 AD), a famous Italian surgeon, wrote and illustrated extensively on exercise and manipulation procedures in medicine.[4] In 18 of his 97 surviving theses, Galen comments on the work of Hippocrates, with illustrations of many of his manipulative techniques.[5]

1.4: Middle Ages and Renaissance Periods

The methods described by Hippocrates and refined by Galen continued to be used throughout the Middle Ages. There was a significant decline in medical knowledge throughout the western world (Europe) and this was largely because the church became responsible for most healing.[3] In medieval Europe, the most common medical practitioners were the barber surgeons who were generally charged with looking after soldiers during or after a battle. These barber surgeons would travel from village to village and provide services from cutting hair to pulling teeth and amputating limbs (Figure 1.4a). They also provided manipulative treatments to reset fractures and became known later as 'bonesetters.' These medieval practitioners of medicine had very little knowledge of the true workings of the human body, as human dissection was prohibited by the church until the 14th century.[6] Between 1506 and 1752, only a limited number of human cadavers were available for dissection for anatomical research, as it was strictly limited to a small number of executed criminals. Around this time, in the Renaissance era, Ambroise Pare (1510-1590) emerged as a famous French physician and barber surgeon. He is credited with using manipulation and traction techniques like those of Hippocrates.

The barber surgeons or bonesetters continued to flourish in Europe from the 1600s through to the late 1800s. In 1656, Friar Thomas Moulton of the Order of St. Augustine published *The Compleat Bone-Setter*. No formal training was required for barber surgeons and bonesetters. The techniques were often learned from family members (apprenticeships) and passed down from one generation to the next.

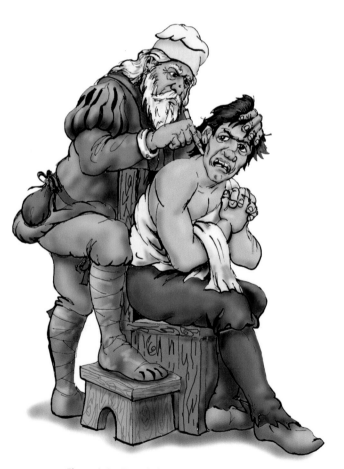

Figure 1.4a: From haircuts to hangnails – the Barber-Surgeon.

1.5: Dawn of Modern Medicine

As barber-surgeons continued their work into the 1700s, the more academically trained surgeons and physicians began to practice more careful observation and scientific method in medicine. John Hunter (1728-1793), a distinguished Scottish surgeon, wrote of the importance of movement of joints after injury for the prevention of stiffness and adhesions. Many other physicians and surgeons in that era would contribute to growing medical knowledge. The proclamation in 1842 by John Evans Riadore (1826-1861) was of interest in that it proposed that anatomical structures (organs) needed adequate neural and vascular supply to sustain health. Riadore advocated the use of manipulation to restore any compromised vascular and neural supply to the body. Subsequently, this concept would be mirrored later in the century by the founders of osteopathy and chiropractic.

Manipulation fell out of favor in medicine when Sir Percival Pott (1714-1788) in describing tuberculosis of the spine (Pott's disease) condemned traction and manipulation as not only useless but dangerous.[3] Despite this, manipulation in the form of bone setting continued to be practiced by lay practitioners and many gained notoriety, such as Mrs. Sarah Mapp (1706-1737). She was apparently so cross-eyed, hideously ugly and fat that she called herself "Crazy Sally" or "Cross-eyed Sally."[7] Although ridiculed by medical society as 'quacks,' many of these bonesetters were much sought after because of the relief they provided to their patients. The realization that orthodox medical practitioners were missing something in the care of their patients led to the publication of a letter by Edward Harrison in 1821 in the *London Medical and Physical Journal*. He proposed that there was a pathophysiologic connection between spinal subluxations and visceral disease. He adjusted vertebrae by pressing on the spinous or transverse processes with his thumbs or with a device.[8] Later, in 1828, Glasgow physician Thomas Brown popularized in the medical community the concept of "spinal irritation." Ultimately, there was the publication of *On Bone-Setting* in 1871 by Wharton Hood[9] in *The Lancet Journal*. Hood learned about bone setting after his father had treated a bonesetter, Richard Hutton.

Hutton was apparently grateful for the medical care and offered to teach his practitioner about bone setting, but it was the practitioner's son, Wharton Hood, who accepted the offer. Hood suggested that the popping or cracking sound with manipulation was the result of breaking joint adhesions, and not that of bones going back into place. Around this time, manipulation was firmly established in contemporary medicine. Many thought that orthodox medicine should consider the adoption of what was good and useful about manipulation but should avoid what was potentially dangerous and useless. An interesting point to note was that manipulation was generally accepted by the medical community some four years before the founding of osteopathy and 28 years before the founding of chiropractic in the United States.

1.6: The Founding of Osteopathy

Osteopathy was founded by Andrew Taylor Still (1826-1917) in 1874 (Figure 1.6a). Still was considered an eccentric nonconformist who garnered considerable wrath among his medical contemporaries. Like his father before him, Still became a physician after completing his formal medical training at the Physicians and Surgeons College of Medicine in Kansas City, Missouri. He practiced orthodox medicine but apparently became disenchanted with it during the Civil War. Some of the medicines commonly given to patients during this time were arsenic, castor oil, whiskey and opium, and unsanitary surgical practices often resulted in more deaths than cures.[10] When his wife and several of his children died from an epidemic of spinal meningitis in 1864, he concluded that the orthodox medical practices of his day were frequently ineffective and sometimes harmful. So, he devoted the next 30 years of his life to studying the human body and finding alternative ways to treat disease. He began investigating alternative treatments such as hydrotherapy, diet, bone setting, and magnetic healing as the relatively tame side effects of those modalities were appealing to him. Thus, he proposed a more rational medical approach that consisted of manipulation of the musculoskeletal system, surgery and very limited use of drugs. He is credited with inventing the name **osteopathy** in 1874 by blending two Greek roots – *osteon* for bone and *pathos* for suffering – to communicate his theory that disease and physiologic dysfunction were etiologically grounded in a disordered musculoskeletal system.

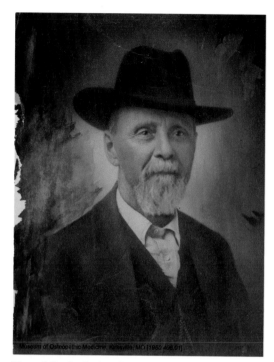

Figure 1.6a: Dr. Andrew Taylor Still, Founder of Osteopathy (Museum of Osteopathic Medicine, Kirksville, MO [1980.406.01]).

In 1892, the first school of osteopathy was formed in Kirksville, Missouri.[11] Among many things, Still proposed that osteopathy was based on the "rule of the artery." His premise was that the body had an innate ability to heal. He further proposed that manipulation could be applied to correct the structural alignment of the spine, thereby allowing blood to flow to various regions of the body to restore the body's homeostasis and natural healing abilities.

The osteopathic profession of today continues to include manipulation in the course curriculum but no longer adheres to Still's original treatment philosophy.[11] Many osteopathic physicians in the United States do not practice manipulation regularly because they are focused on allopathic specialty areas, such as internal medicine or emergency medicine.

1.7: The Founding of Chiropractic

Chiropractic was founded in 1895 by Daniel David Palmer (1845-1913) (Figure 1.7a). Palmer was a former green grocer, school teacher and a practicing "magnetic healer." According to legend, in 1895, while working as a magnetic healer in Davenport, Iowa, he encountered the building's janitor whose hearing was severely impaired. Palmer discovered a palpable lump in the janitor's back and theorized that this lump and the hearing deficits were related. He manipulated the thoracic spine and claimed to successfully restore the man's hearing.

Palmer's theories revolved around the concept that altered nerve flow was the cause of all disease, and that misalignment of spinal vertebrae had an effect on that nerve flow. He postulated that restoring these vertebrae to their correct alignment would restore health. His writings include, "A subluxated vertebra … is the cause of 95 percent of all diseases…The other five percent is caused by displaced joints other than those of the vertebral column."

In 1896, Palmer's first descriptions and underlying philosophy of chiropractic was strikingly similar to Andrew Taylor Still's principles of osteopathy established a decade earlier.[12] Both described the body as a "machine" whose parts could be manipulated to correct misalignments and produce a drugless cure. The chiropractors called these misalignments a "subluxation" which interfered with the nervous system while the osteopaths dubbed them as "somatic dysfunction" which affected the circulatory system. Soon after, osteopaths began an American-wide campaign to proclaim that chiropractic was a bastardized form of osteopathy and sought licensure to differentiate the two groups.[12] Although Palmer initially denied being trained by osteopathic medicine founder A.T. Still, in 1899 in papers held at the Palmer College of Chiropractic, he wrote:

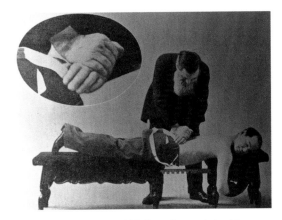

Figure 1.7a: Daniel David Palmer demonstrates his chiropractic method of spinal adjustments, designed to alleviate pressure on the nerves that he believed caused disease (Courtesy of Special Collections and Archives, Palmer College of Chiropractic).

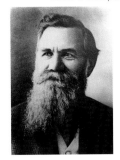

"Some years ago I took an expensive course in Electropathy, Cranial Diagnosis, Hydrotherapy, Facial Diagnosis. Later I took Osteopathy [which] gave me such a measure of confidence as to almost feel it unnecessary to seek other sciences for the mastery of curable disease. Having been assured that the underlying philosophy of chiropractic is the same as that of osteopathy…Chiropractic is osteopathy gone to seed."[13]

One of the first graduates of the Palmer School of Chiropractic in Davenport, Iowa, was Palmer's son Bartlett Joshua Palmer (1882-1961), who later ran the school and promoted the growth of the profession. Although practitioners of the traditional (straight) chiropractic theory have declined in more recent times, these concepts persist as the primary teaching emphasis in several existing chiropractic schools. These "straight" chiropractors continue to adhere to Palmer's original subluxation theories and use spinal adjustments as the primary means of treatment. Most chiropractors today could be referred to as "mixers," in that they incorporate other rehabilitative interventions into the treatment options, including physical modalities, such as therapeutic ultrasound, electrical stimulation and exercise.

1.8: Early Physical Therapy

In 1867, the *British Medical Journal* reported on a lecture by Dr. James Paget, *"On the Cases that Bonesetters Cure."*[14] As previously noted, in 1871, Dr. Wharton Hood wrote a series complementary to bone setting for the *Lancet* based on his experiences with a bonesetter named Richard Hutton.[9,15] Also, in 1882, bone setting was the main topic at the 50th annual meeting of the British Medical Association's Section on Surgery in Worcester England in August.[16] These times saw a renewed interest in manual or physical therapy interventions. This may have been because of the influx and successful establishment of thriving practices by the earliest Swedish-educated physical therapists in various countries, including the United Kingdom. Physical Therapy as a government-sanctioned, university-educated profession began in 1813, when Pehr Hendrik Ling (1776 -1839) founded the Kungliga Gymnastiska Centralinstitutet or Royal Central Institute for Gymnastics (RCIG) in Stockholm.[17] Students at the RCIG were either noblemen or belonged to the upper echelons of society. Most were also army officers. Ling's educational system included four branches: pedagogical gymnastics (physical education), military gymnastics (mostly fencing), medical gymnastics (physical therapy), and esthetic gymnastics (philosophy). The medical gymnastics taught and practiced included a strong manual therapy component. Although by today's standards, the manual therapy component instructed in Ling's system can hardly be called segment specific (Figure 1.8a).

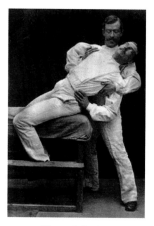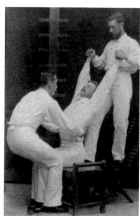

Figure 1.8a: Lumbar (left) and thoracic (right) manipulation as per Ling.

However, clinicians educated at the RCIG certainly further developed and published more specific manipulative interventions.

While Ling may not be credited as the originator of medical gymnastics or massage, he certainly systematized these methods and attempted to add contemporary knowledge of anatomy and physiology to support medical gymnastics. Ling put forth his "doctrine of harmony" purporting that the health of the body depended on the balance between three primary forms: mechanics (movement/exercise/manipulation), chemistry (food/medicine), and dynamics (psychiatry). Just as osteopathy and chiropractic would do in the future, the Ling physical therapists were trained in the 1830s to restore this harmony through use of manual therapy, including manipulation, in clinics in many European cities.

Around this time in Sweden, an 80-year turf war erupted between these early physical therapists and the fledgling orthopedic medicine specialization from which the orthopedic physicians at the Karolinska Institute eventually emerged victorious.[18,19] Consequently, physical therapy education in Sweden and eventually the rest of the world was restructured to a technical education producing allied health technicians. In English-language countries, physical therapy was soon practiced by nurses with additional course work in massage and exercise therapy. In other Western European countries, physical education teachers with additional course work in rehabilitative exercise gave up their previous professional independence, often begrudgingly, for support from the medical profession in their search for societal recognition.[19]

Soon after this, national associations were created by these physical therapy technicians. In 1889 in the Netherlands, physical therapists founded the world's first professional association, the Society for Practicing Heilgymnastics in the Netherlands. In 1894, in Great Britain, the Society of Trained Masseuses was founded, and in 1906 in Australia, the Australasian Massage Association.[19,20] Physical therapy in the United States had a somewhat later start as the founding of the American Women's Physical Therapeutic Association did not occur until 1921. Once embroiled in World War I, the US did not, in contrast to its European allies, have a military with an established division of physical therapy. The Surgeon General, to remedy this, commanded that several university physical education programs should institute physiotherapy "War Emergency Courses" to train women who would be able to physically rehabilitate returning soldiers.

When, in 1922, the military reduced therapy services because of government cutbacks, many therapists previously employed by the military were forced into the private sector. This led to conflicts with other manual therapy practitioners including nurses, osteopaths, and chiropractors all claiming to practice physical therapy. It was this early conflict, especially with the chiropractic profession, that caused physical therapists to align themselves more closely with medical physicians. In 1930, to garner physician support, the U.S. physical therapists voluntarily relinquished their right to see patients without physician referral.[21]

Because of the close alliance with the medical physicians and the adversarial relationship between physicians and chiropractors, physical therapists tended to deemphasize the use of manual therapy in their clinical practice. However, these interventions continued to be used and further developed within the profession with various publications during this period in the US professional physical therapy literature.[22] In Western Europe, Scandinavia and Australasia, this adversarial stance never developed. Instead, medical physicians embraced manual therapy approaches and postgraduate manual medicine training institutes were well-attended by physicians. Several prominent European orthopedic physicians influenced the practice of manipulation and the evolution of the physical therapist's role as a manipulative therapist.

Between 1912 and 1935, James B. Mennell (1880-1957) provided advanced training in manipulation technique for physiotherapists at St. Thomas's Hospital in London. In 1949, Mennell published his textbook titled *The Science and Art of Joint Manipulation*.[23] Dr. Mennell adapted knowledge of joint mechanics in the practice of manipulation and coined the phrase "accessory motion."[23]

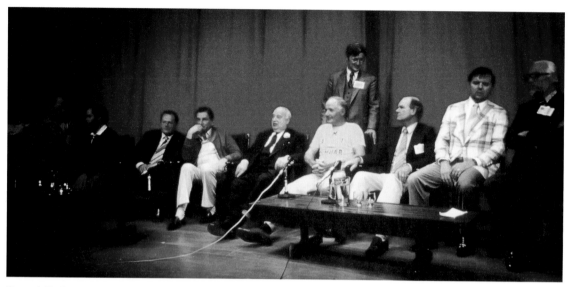

Figure 1.8b: Dr. James H, Cyriax at the 1980 IFOMT General Meeting in Christchurch, New Zealand, with physiotherapists from left: Olaf Evjenth, Richard Erhart, Vladimir Janda, Dr. Schmidt, James Cyriax, Robin McKenzie with Stanley Paris behind, Geoffrey Maitland, Sandy Burkhart, Alan Stoddard.

James H. Cyriax (1904–1985) published his classic *Textbook of Orthopaedic Medicine* in 1954. He made great contributions to orthopedic medicine with the development of detailed systematic examination procedures for extremity disorders. This included refinement of isometric tissue tension signs, end feel assessment, and capsular patterns.[24] Dr. Cyriax attributed most back pain to disorders of the intervertebral disc and used aggressive general manipulation techniques that included strong manual traction forces to "reduce the disc." Dr. Cyriax, who also taught and practiced orthopedic medicine at St. Thomas's Hospital until 1969, influenced many physiotherapists to carry on the skills and techniques required to effectively use manipulation (Figure 1.8b). He is reported to have stated that physical therapists were the most apt professionals to learn manipulative techniques.[21]

Another influential person teaching manipulation to physical therapists at the time, at the London School of Osteopathy, was Dr. Alan Stoddard (1915–2002). Dr. Stoddard was a medical and osteopathic physician in England who used skillful specific manipulation technique mentoring many physical therapists.

1.9: Manual Therapy Approaches

In the 1960s, several physical therapists emerged as international leaders in the practice and instruction of manipulation. Physical therapist Freddy Kaltenborn, originally from Norway, was trained as a physical education teacher when he was admitted as the first male student to the Norwegian program in physical therapy in 1948. Educated in London in orthopedic medicine by Dr. James Cyriax from 1952 to 1954, he qualified in chiropractic in Germany in 1958 and in osteopathy at the London School of Osteopathy with Dr. Stoddard in 1962. Kaltenborn was soon associated with physical therapist Olav Evjenth. Together, they developed an eclectic manual therapy system known as the Kaltenborn-Evjenth approach. He published his first textbook on spinal manipulation in 1964 and was the first to relate manipulation to arthrokinematics. His techniques were specific and perpetuated the importance of biomechanical principles, such as the concave/convex and arthrokinematic rules. In collaboration with Evjenth, he also developed extensive long-term training programs for physical therapists to specialize in manual therapy, first in Norway and later throughout Europe, North America, and Asia.

Australian physical therapist Geoffrey Maitland (1924-2010), after studying abroad with Dr. Cyriax and Dr. Stoddard, and physical therapists Gregory Grieve and Jennifer Hickling, developed his own approach and started teaching his manual therapy system at the University of Adelaide in South Australia. This was done initially in the entry-level physical therapy program. He went on to develop 12-month postgraduate diploma courses in manipulative therapy which were offered at physical therapy programs in Australia. Maitland published the first edition of his textbook, *Vertebral Manipulation*, in 1964 around the same time as Kaltenborn's first textbook. Maitland is credited with further refining the importance of a detailed history and comprehensive physical examination. He also developed the concept of treatment of "reproducible signs" and inhibition of joint pain with use of gentle oscillatory mobilization techniques. Somewhat unique to the Maitland approach was the concept of frequent, immediate post-intervention reevaluations of the deemed most concordant (or so-called 'asterisk' signs) to guide further management.

The differences between the Kaltenborn/Evjenth and Maitland approaches resulted in some competitive but 'friendly rivalry' between the two philosophies, which continues to exist today to some degree. However, the eclectic evolution of orthopaedic manual therapy allows more than enough room to accommodate both. The differences are irrelevant historically. However, what is more important to note is that, together, they underscore the essence of physical therapy's role in the advancement of joint manipulation. In the technically skilled hands of a physical therapist, advancements in medical science have been translated into safer, more effective manipulative techniques.[25]

Also in the early 1960s, physical therapist Stanley Paris from New Zealand received a scholarship to study manipulation with Dr. Cyriax, Kaltenborn and Dr. Stoddard in Europe. On his return to New Zealand, he organized courses and introduced, among others, influential physical therapists Robin McKenzie and Brian Mulligan to manual therapy before leaving to teach and practice in the United States. Paris became the voice of manual therapy as a specialization within orthopedic physical therapy within the United States and worldwide.

As orthopedic manual therapy grew around the world, there were calls for the formation of a central organization. During the World Confederation of Physical Therapy (WCPT) conference in Denmark in 1970, a group of therapists were tasked with working with the WCPT to create its first sub-group, the International Federation of Orthopaedic Manipulative Therapists (IFOMT). The committee and consultants included McKenzie, Paris, Kaltenborn, Grieve, David Lamb, and Maitland. IFOMT was founded in Montreal in 1974, and with it came the recommendations of standards and the setting of examinations to allow physical therapists entry into the newly formed organization.

In 1991, eight physical therapists; Dick Erhard, Joe Farrell, Ola Grimsby, Kornelia Kulig, Michael Moore, Stanley Paris, Mike Rogers and Bjorn Swensen, founded the American Academy of Orthopedic Manual Therapy (AAOMPT). Farrell was elected the first president of the academy and presided over the Academy's first meeting in Las Vegas. Prior to this time, there was no organization in the United States that was dedicated to the promotion and education of manual therapy. AAOMPT was formed for several reasons. First, it was felt that post-graduate training (e.g. residency and fellowship training) in orthopedic manual physical therapy required an accreditation process to ensure that a high level of education standards was established in the US. Secondly, it wanted to provide pathways for discussion, education and research in orthopedic manual physical therapy. Thirdly, it was created to become a member country of IFOMT.

Farrell, Carol Jo Tichenor and Kornelia Kulig prepared the application for US membership in IFOMT. The educational standards from this document formed the basis for the AAOMPT Standards Committee review process of manual therapy fellowships, which then contributed to the current accreditation process of the American Board of Physical Therapy Residency and Fellowship Education (ABPTRFE). In 1996, AAOMPT opened Fellowship challenge through portfolio by experienced therapists who had not gone through formal residencies but had extensive experience in manual therapy. The portfolios included video tapes of these individuals with live patients, documenting experience in teaching and training.

In 1998, AAOMPT Board of Directors approved an additional pathway to challenge for fellowship through examination. Using the original template established by Mike Rogers, Kornelia Kulig, Bjorn Swenson and Dick Erhard to examine each other's program, they established the initial challenge examinations by Objective Structured Clinical Examination (OSCE). Dick Erhard, Katherine Patla, Bjorn Swenson and Bill O'Grady were chosen to be the original examiners in Boston and Denver. In 2001-2002, the chair of the examination committee, O'Grady, and his committee conducted the largest scale oral practical examination to date, examining a total of 49 candidates in both Orlando and at the University of Pittsburgh Medical Center. Mike Puniello, his successor, continued these examinations for an additional two years. The testing was discontinued in 2004 as the Academy moved to have the primary pathway to fellowship be through formal residency/ fellowship training.

When all of this was taking place early in the development of AAOMPT, Farrell was serving as a Director of the Orthopaedic Section of the APTA. AAOMPT and the Orthopaedic Sections Board of Directors, at Steve McDavitt's (Orthopaedic Section practice affairs chair) urging, organized the APTA National Manipulation Strategic Planning meeting in Washington, DC (1999) to develop an evidence-based plan of action to deal with the chronic battles with chiropractors over the scope of physical therapy practice. Farrell organized this strategic meeting, while McDavitt was the meeting facilitator of the participants which included clinicians, academic faculty, researchers, APTA staff and lobbyists. The outcome of the meeting convinced the APTA to develop a long-term plan of action to protect clinical practice as outlined in the Guide to Physical Therapy Practice. From this 1999 meeting, the APTA Manipulation Task Force was developed, which in turn formulated an action template which has been invaluable to many state chapters and individuals who have faced legal and legislative challenges in reference to practice infringement (e.g. from chiropractors, athletic trainers, personal trainers, massage therapists, etc.). Recently, resources developed by the original Manipulation Task Force were utilized to restore manipulation as a component of the Washington State Practice Act (2015) and by the Georgia APTA chapter for their successful legislative effort to modernize their Physical Therapy Practice Act in 2015.

Although prominent individuals have played a large role in the development and advancement of manipulation and manual therapy within the physical therapy profession over the last half of the twentieth century, the current practice and the future of the specialty area of orthopaedic manual physical therapy are driven by evidence-based practice. The continued promotion of orthopaedic manual physical therapy practice has been through professional associations, such as IFOMT, AAOMPT, and the APTA. A large and growing body of research evidence supports and guides the practice of manipulation within the scope of physical therapy practice and for other manual therapy practitioners.

1.10: Key Points from Chapter 1

- Spinal manipulation has been practiced for the relief of symptoms for many centuries.
- Many different practitioners have provided spinal manipulation over those centuries.
- Currently, spinal manipulation is practiced by many different professionals, including physical therapists.
- Much of the recent research into the safety and efficacy of spinal manipulation has been conducted by physical therapists.

Chapter 1 References

1. Hippocrates. *The Genuine Works of Hippocrates.* Baltimore, MD: Williams & Wilkins; 1939.
2. Lewit K. *Manipulative Therapy: Musculoskeletal Medicine.* Elsevier; 2010.
3. Paris SV. A History of Manipulative Therapy Through the Ages and Up to the Current Controversy in the United States. *Journal of Manual & Manipulative Therapy.* 2000;8(2):66-77.
4. Galen C. Galen: *Method of Medicine, Volume I: Books 1-4 (Loeb Classical Library).* Vol 1. Boston, MA: Harvard University Press; 2011.
5. Paris SV. Historical Perspectives in Orthopaedic Manual Physical Therapy. In: Wise C, ed. *Orthopaedic Manual Physical Therapy.* Philadelphia, PA: F.A. Davis Company; 2015.
6. Grauer A. *A Companion to Paleopathology.* John Wiley & Sons; 2011.
7. Pownall H. Mrs Mapp The Female Bone-setter. 2015; http://www.epsomandewellhistoryexplorer.org.uk/MappMrs.html. Accessed November 2015.
8. Weiner MF, Silver JR. Edward Harrison and the treatment of spinal deformities in the nineteenth century. *J R Coll Physicians Edinb.* 2008;38(3):265-271.
9. Hood W. On Bone-Setting. *The Lancet.* 1871;97(2488):631.
10. Hansen GP. Beyond OMT: time for a new chapter in osteopathic medicine? *J Am Osteopath Assoc.* 2006;106(3):114-116.
11. Miller K. The evolution of professional identity: the case of osteopathic medicine. *Soc Sci Med.* 1998;47(11):1739-1748.
12. Ernst E. Chiropractic: a critical evaluation. *J Pain Symptom Manage.* 2008;35(5):544-562.
13. Leach R. *The Chiropractic Theories: A Textbook of Scientific Research.* Lippincott, Williams and Wilkins; 2004.
14. Paget J. Clinical Lecture on Cases that Bone-Setters Cure. *Br Med J.* 1867;1(314):1-4.
15. Hood W. On the so-called "Bone-Setting", its nature and results. *The Lancet.* 1871;97(2480):336-338.
16. Prichard A. The Address Delivered in the Section of Surgery. *Br Med J.* 1882;2(1128):263-265.
17. Brodin H. [Per Henrik Ling and his impact on gymnastics]. *Sven Med Tidskr.* 2008;12(1):61-68.
18. A. O. *Sjukgymnasten-Vart Tog Han Vägen?* Göteborg, Sweden: Historiska Institutionen Göteborgs Universitet 2005.
19. Kaltenborn F. Early history of physiotherapy in Sweden and Norway: Implications for professional autonomy and direct-access clinical practice. *Tijdschrift Manuele Therapie.* 2008;5(2):6-9.
20. Terlouw TJA. Roots of Physical Medicine, Physical Therapy, and Mechanotherapy in the Netherlands in the 19th Century: A Disputed Area within the Healthcare Domain. *Journal of Manual & Manipulative Therapy.* 2007;15(2):23E-41E.
21. Huijbregts PA. Chiropractic Legal Challenges to the Physical Therapy Scope of Practice: Anybody Else Taking the Ethical High Ground? *Journal of Manual & Manipulative Therapy.* 2007;15(2):69-80.
22. Linker B. Strength and Science: Gender, Physiotherapy, and Medicine in the United States, 1918-35. *Journal of Women's History* 2005;17(3):106-132.
23. Mennell J. *The science and art of joint manipulation.* London: J. & A. Churchill Ltd.; 1949.
24. Cyriax JH. *Textbook of Oerthopaedic Medicine. Vol I, Diagnosis of Soft Tissue Lesions.* London: Cassell; 1954.
25. Pettman E. *A History of Manipulative Therapy. The Journal of Manual & Manipulative Therapy.* 2007;15(3):165-174.

Chapter 2

Evidence for the Use of Thrust Joint Manipulation

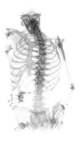

2.1: Chapter Objectives

When considering the use of thrust joint manipulation (TJM) in the management of a patient's spinal dysfunction, clinicians are encouraged to practice in an evidence-based or, perhaps, evidence-informed manner. All the manual therapy professions recognize that evidence-based practice is central to providing high-quality care and decreasing unwarranted variation in clinical practice. Evidence-based practice is defined as "the integration of best available research, clinical expertise, and patient values and circumstances related to patient and client management, practice management and health policy decision-making"[1] (Figure 2.1a).

So, what does the best available research evidence for the use of TJM tell us? To answer this appropriately, we must first be able to critically appraise the available research evidence. In this chapter, we will critically appraise the current research evidence for, and against, TJM in the management of spinal pain and dysfunction. We will argue that much of the research evidence may well be fatally flawed by the use of heterogeneous sampling (all patients/subjects with spinal pain) and poorly defined/controlled experimental interventions (TJM).

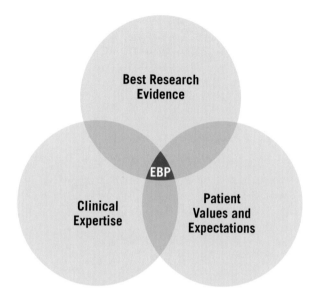

Figure 2.1a: Evidence-Based Practice seen as the intersection of best available research evidence, clinical expertise, and patient values and expectations.

2.2: The Hierarchy of Evidence: What is the "Best Evidence"?

The hierarchy of evidence is a core principal of evidence-based practice and attempts to answer the question, "What is the best available evidence"? These hierarchies will typically rank the differing study types based on the rigor of their research methods. Most experts will agree that the higher up the hierarchal pyramid a study is positioned, the more rigorous the methodology and hence, the more likely it is that the results of the study can be trusted in clinical practice. In most evidence hierarchies current, well-designed systematic reviews and meta-analyses will be found at the top of the pyramid, and expert opinion and anecdotal experience are at the bottom[2] (Figure 2.2a). However, different hierarchies exist for different research question types and even experts may disagree on the exact rank of information in the various evidence hierarchies.

One particularly amusing study may help to illustrate the importance of understanding or appraising the available research evidence. Smith and Pell[3] observed that parachutes are used in recreational, voluntary sector, and military settings to reduce the risk of orthopedic, head, and soft tissue injuries following gravitational challenges, such as jumping from an aircraft in flight. They suggested that the perception that parachutes are a successful intervention is based largely on anecdotal evidence. Therefore, they sought to determine whether parachutes are effective in preventing major trauma related to gravitational challenge. They conducted a systematic review of randomized controlled trials involving parachutes as interventions, and, not surprisingly, found that there were none.[3] They concluded that, like many other interventions intended to treat or prevent ill health, the effectiveness of parachutes has not been subject to rigorous evaluation by using randomized controlled trials.[3] With tongue very much in cheek, they proposed two options. The first was that clinicians accept that, under exceptional circumstances, common sense might be applied when considering potential risks and benefits of interventions.[3] The second was that clinicians continue their 'quest for the holy grail of exclusively evidence-based interventions' and preclude parachute use outside the context of a properly conducted trial.[3] Hilariously, they then suggested that those who advocate evidence-based medicine and criticize use of interventions that lack an evidence base should demonstrate their commitment by volunteering for a double-blind, randomized, placebo-controlled, crossover trial!

With their publication in the *British Medical Journal*, Smith and Pell[3] made the excellent point that evidence-based practice should not focus solely on best research evidence at the exclusion of clinical expertise (common sense) and patient values and expectations.

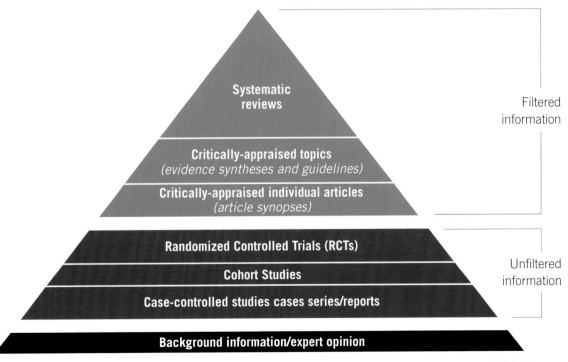

Figure 2.2a: The hierarchy of evidence provided by the Australian National Health and Medical Research Council (NHMRC).

2.3: Evidence for Thrust Joint Manipulation in the Lumbar Spine – Systematic Reviews

As systematic reviews are considered the 'top of the evidence pyramid,' we will begin by analyzing some recent ones. In 2017, Rothberg and Friedman[4] published the results of their systematic review of complementary therapies in addition to medication for patients with non-chronic, non-radicular low back pain. Their narrow focus was on randomized studies that included patients with non-radicular low back pain (LBP) of less than 12 weeks' duration that compared spinal manipulative therapy to usual care, sham therapy, or interventions known not to be efficacious, while providing all patients with standard analgesics (medical therapy).

They found only two randomized controlled trials in which TJM in addition to medical therapy failed to show any benefit when compared to medical therapy alone.[4] On the strength of their findings from only two studies, they concluded that, for patients with non-chronic, non-radicular LBP, available evidence does not support the use of TJM in addition to standard medical therapy.[4] It is remarkable that the authors could draw such definitive conclusions from only two studies, especially when a review of those studies[5] shows that the intervention of interest (TJM) was not actually provided to all subjects in the two studies. One study provided spinal manipulative therapy "according to a treatment algorithm developed by the researchers on the basis of views of expert clinicians and researchers"[5] which permitted the use of non-thrust mobilization *or* high-velocity thrust joint manipulation. Their results show that TJM was only provided on 12 out of 239 treatment sessions (five percent).[5] The second study defined spinal manipulative therapy as "a combination of high-velocity low-amplitude thrusts, spinal mobilizations and muscle energy techniques"[6] which again permitted the use of either non-thrust joint mobilization or high-velocity TJM. Their results show that TJM was applied in an estimated 80 percent of all sessions, to at least 73 percent of the patients allocated to the manipulation group.[6] In both studies, the intervention being studied (TJM) was not provided consistently, and therefore, it may not be surprising to see little to no difference between groups.

In 2016, Ruddock et al[7] published the results of their systematic review and meta-analysis of spinal manipulation versus sham manipulation for non-specific LBP. They noted that previous reviews had compared spinal manipulation to sham manipulations; however, they had either included articles that did not use an effective sham[8] or permitted techniques that were not solely TJM.[8-11] For their review, the authors clearly stated their purpose was to assess TJM in isolation rather than as part of a treatment package of care, so that any specific treatment effects could be isolated to TJM. To be eligible for the review, studies also had to use an effective sham intervention for the comparison group.[7]

They found nine randomized studies which could be included in the systematic review, and four were eligible for meta-analysis. Results showed that participants in the spinal manipulation group had improved symptoms compared with those receiving sham treatment (standard mean difference = -0.36; 95% CI = -0.59 to -0.12)[7] (Figure 2.3a). They concluded that there was some evidence that spinal TJM has specific treatment effects and is more effective at reducing non-specific LBP when compared with an effective sham intervention. The effect size was found to be small to medium in terms of clinical relevance; however, the included studies had rather broad inclusion criteria where participants could have had symptom duration anywhere between less than 48 hours[12] to greater than six months.[13] All practicing clinicians would concede that spinal TJM is not effective for all patients with non-specific LBP, and the inclusion of participants less likely to benefit from it (perhaps those with longer duration of symptoms) could have masked the true effect size in terms of clinical relevance.

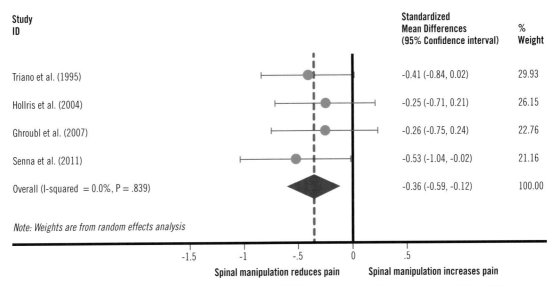

Study ID		Standardized Mean Differences (95% Confidence interval)	% Weight
Triano et al. (1995)		-0.41 (-0.84, 0.02)	29.93
Hollris et al. (2004)		-0.25 (-0.71, 0.21)	26.15
Ghroubl et al. (2007)		-0.26 (-0.75, 0.24)	22.76
Senna et al. (2011)		-0.53 (-1.04, -0.02)	21.16
Overall (I-squared = 0.0%, P = .839)		-0.36 (-0.59, -0.12)	100.00

Note: Weights are from random effects analysis

-1.5   -1   -.5   0   .5

Spinal manipulation reduces pain   **Spinal manipulation increases pain**

Figure 2.3a: Forest plot of the meta-analysis of pain scores of 287 participants receiving spinal manipulation (SM) versus sham spinal manipulation. Adapted from Ruddock et al.[7]

In 2014, Merepeza[14] published the results of a systematic review comparing the effects of spinal manipulation versus therapeutic exercise on adults with chronic LBP. An inclusion criterion for studies was that patients had to have low back pain persisting 12 weeks or longer.[14] Only three studies were included in the review, with one finding spinal manipulation to be more effective than exercise, a second finding exercises to be more effective than spinal manipulation, and the third study finding no difference between the interventions.[14] Although study participants could be said to be a homogeneous sampling of people with LBP of at least 12 weeks duration, the intervention investigated (spinal manipulation) was not standardized. Two studies defined spinal manipulation as "mobilization *and/or* manipulation"[15,16] and the third defined it as "manual procedures,"[17] so it could be argued that spinal TJM was not truly evaluated as the intervention of interest.

Finally, in the most recently published systematic review, Paige et al[18] studied the effectiveness of spinal manipulative therapy for acute (≤ 6 weeks) low back pain. Out of 26 eligible studies, 15 randomized controlled trials involving 1,711 patients provided moderate quality evidence that manipulation has a statistically significant association with improvements in pain.[18] For pain, the pooled mean improvement in the 100-mm visual analog pain scale was only 9.95 mm (95% CI = 4.3 – 15.6).[18] This does not meet or exceed the minimal detectable change for LBP of 20 mm, nor the minimal clinically important difference of 22 mm.[19] They also found moderate quality evidence from 12 trials involving 1,381 patients that manipulation has a statistically significant association with improvements in function.[18] For measures of disability, mean pooled effect size was 0.39 (95% CI = 0.07 – 0.71),[18] which represents a medium effect size.[20] This review is important because they limited meta-analysis to patients with acute LBP which they defined as ≤ 6 weeks. Also, some attempt was made to classify the spinal manipulative therapy. The authors included studies that provided either thrust *or* non-thrust manipulation, but did exclude studies where the intervention could not be classified. We could speculate that results may have been different if only studies that provided TJM had been included. However, direct evidence that different kinds of manipulation have different efficacy is still lacking.[18]

2.4: Evidence for Thrust Joint Manipulation in the Lumbar Spine – Randomized Controlled Trials

There is a wealth of published research on TJM clinical trials for LBP. We performed a quick internet search using the terms "evidence" AND "manipulation" AND "low back pain" AND "clinical trials" and found 4,040 results. One of the most widely-read and discussed studies was the United Kingdom Back Pain Exercise and Manipulation (UK BEAM) clinical trial.[21] This particular clinical trial involved 181 general medical practices in 63 community settings around 14 centers across the United Kingdom, and 1,334 patients consulting their general practitioners about LBP.[21] Patients were randomized into four groups: usual (best) care, exercise plus usual care, manipulation plus usual care, or manipulation and exercise plus usual care; and outcome measures were collected at baseline, three months, and one year via questionnaires. At baseline, the mean (SD) age of patients was 43 (11) years; 56 percent were female; more than half had had pain for more than 90 days; and the mean (SD) Roland-Morris Disability Questionnaire score was 9.0 (4.0) out of a possible 24 points. Results showed that all four groups demonstrated statistically significant differences from baseline (Figure 2.4a). However, only the manipulation and manipulation plus exercise groups demonstrated changes beyond the minimal clinically important difference of 3.5 points.[22]

It is important to consider two issues with this study. First, no attempt was made to sub-group patients with low back pain, and so the sample of 1,334 patients was heterogeneous in terms of symptom duration, with 58.7 percent reporting pain > 90 days. Secondly, the 'manipulation' provided in the study was a 'package of techniques' representative of those used by the UK chiropractic, osteopathic and physiotherapy professions.[23] These techniques represented a 'pragmatic' rather than a prescriptive approach. As a result, TJM was not provided consistently and, in fact, only had to be provided 'at least once.'[21] It would be interesting to see what would result from a repeat study that used a more homogeneous sample of patients with LBP, and all subjects in the manipulation group actually received TJM every time they received treatment interventions.

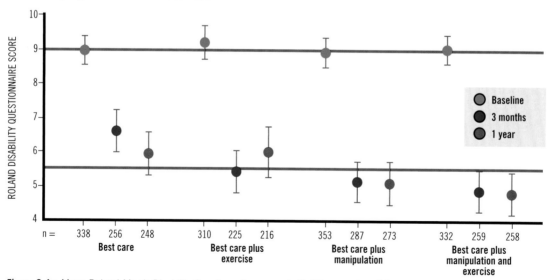

Figure 2.4a: Mean Roland-Morris Disability Questionnaire scores (with 95 percent confidence intervals) over 12 months by group: best care in general practice, best care plus exercise alone, best care plus manipulation alone, and best care plus manipulation and exercise. The red lines indicate the Minimal Clinically Important Difference (MCID) of 3.5 points from the baseline mean of 9.0. Adapted from UK Beam Trial Team.[21]

In a follow-up study, the UK Beam Trial Team explored the views of participants in the trial about the treatment packages they received.[24] They collected a total of 1,259 comments from 1,334 study participants, and those randomized to receive manipulation felt the intervention was appropriate to their needs and commonly reported striking benefits.[24] The authors concluded that the qualitative analysis found much clearer differences between the groups than the main quantitative analysis.

Hurwitz et al[25] conducted a randomized controlled trial of chiropractic and medical care for patients with LBP with 18-month follow-up as part of the University of California Los Angeles (UCLA) LBP study. A total of 681 patients with LBP presenting to a managed-care facility were randomized to receive chiropractic with or without physical modalities, or medical care with or without physical therapy.[25] There were 610 (89.6%) patients at 18-month follow-up for analysis, and results suggested that differences in outcomes between medical and chiropractic care without physical therapy or modalities were not clinically meaningful.[25] Analysis of baseline variables for the study show that 26.1 percent of patients had duration of symptoms < three weeks; 15.6 percent were three weeks to three months; 11.6 percent were three months to one year; and 46.7 percent were > one year. Therefore, there was a heterogeneous sample of acute, sub-acute and chronic LBP. Furthermore, the chiropractic care provided in the study was defined as spinal manipulation *or* mobilization, instruction in strengthening and flexibility exercises, and instruction in proper back care.

Hancock et al[5] conducted a randomized controlled trial of non-steroidal anti-inflammatory medication (diclofenac) versus spinal manipulative therapy in the recovery of patients with acute LBP. They randomly assigned 240 patients with acute LBP (symptom duration less than six weeks) to one of four groups: manipulation plus diclofenac; placebo manipulation plus diclofenac; manipulation plus placebo diclofenac; and placebo manipulation plus placebo diclofenac.[5] The primary outcome measure was total number of days to recovery, which was defined as the number of days it took for patients to report seven consecutive days with a pain score of zero or one out of 10 scale. Results showed that there were no significant differences between groups, and therefore, the authors concluded that neither diclofenac nor spinal manipulative therapy appreciably reduced the number of days to recovery compared with the placebo interventions.[5] While this study did use a relatively homogeneous sample of patients with LBP, the spinal manipulation intervention provided to patients was mostly non-thrust mobilization (97 percent). Only a very small proportion received TJM (five percent). Given this fact, it may not be all that surprising that results were not significantly different between manipulation and placebo manipulation groups.

Cecchi et al[26] compared spinal manipulation, back school and individual physiotherapy in the treatment of chronic LBP. They had 210 patients randomly allocated to a back school group (70); an individual physiotherapy group (70); and a spinal manipulation group (70) and followed them at discharge from therapy at three, six and 12 months. While there were no significant differences for pain ratings across groups at discharge (p = 0.401), there were differences at all other time points in favor of the manipulation group (p < 0.001).[26] Additionally, there were significant differences for disability ratings (Roland-Morris) for all follow-up time points in favor of manipulation (p < 0.001).[26] Patients in the study had mean (SD) of 58.3 (14.4) years, and although no data was provided on mean duration of symptoms, they had to report experiencing non-specific LBP 'often' to 'always' for at least the past six months.[26] However, the spinal manipulation intervention was rather vaguely defined as "consisting of vertebral direct and indirect mobilization and manipulation, with associated soft tissue manipulation, as needed."[26] It is therefore difficult to conclude that spinal manipulation resulted in the observed differences between the patient groups.

When randomized clinical trial designs allow for too much variability in the intervention of interest, one could argue that the study would not truly examine that intervention of interest. When studies purporting to examine the effectiveness of TJM fail to actually provide it as the experimental intervention, we should not be surprised to see non-significant outcomes. Many researchers have argued that allowing for a more pragmatic design in studies can result in more realistic findings that are based on practical rather than theoretical considerations. If clinicians believe that research has investigated cohorts that do not resemble the patients they see, and if they think that the interventions have been implemented in a manner that does not resemble their clinical practice, they are unlikely to adopt recommendations on the basis of that research.[27] This represents a conundrum as effective research requires controlled interventions, whereas clinical practice requires flexibility in the provision of interventions to suit the patient.

Kent et al[27] conducted a systematic review and meta-analysis to test the hypothesis that randomized clinical trials of manual therapy for non-specific LBP would show greater therapeutic effect when participating clinicians were given discretion regarding treatment selection. In other words, would there be better outcomes with pragmatic versus prescriptive study designs? The authors found 10 randomized clinical trials that met their strict inclusion criteria, and calculated effect sizes and performed inverse variance meta-analytic pooling.[27] Clinicians were able to choose their preferred treatment interventions in 70 percent of the included trials, and results showed that pooled estimates of effect size for short-term pain favored the clinical trials where clinicians did not have treatment technique choice[27] (Figure 2.5a). Also, pooled estimates of effect size for short-term activity limitation favored the clinical trials where clinicians did not have treatment technique choice[27] (Figure 2.5b). These findings suggest that allowing participating clinicians' discretion regarding

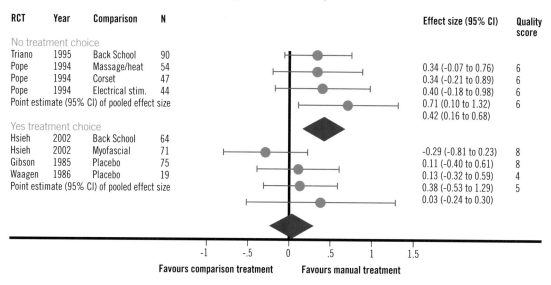

Change in short-term pain

RCT	Year	Comparison	N	Effect size (95% CI)	Quality score
No treatment choice					
Triano	1995	Back School	90	0.34 (-0.07 to 0.76)	6
Pope	1994	Massage/heat	54	0.34 (-0.21 to 0.89)	6
Pope	1994	Corset	47	0.40 (-0.18 to 0.98)	6
Pope	1994	Electrical stim.	44	0.71 (0.10 to 1.32)	6
Point estimate (95% CI) of pooled effect size				0.42 (0.16 to 0.68)	
Yes treatment choice					
Hsieh	2002	Back School	64	-0.29 (-0.81 to 0.23)	8
Hsieh	2002	Myofascial	71	0.11 (-0.40 to 0.61)	8
Gibson	1985	Placebo	75	0.13 (-0.32 to 0.59)	4
Waagen	1986	Placebo	19	0.38 (-0.53 to 1.29)	5
Point estimate (95% CI) of pooled effect size				0.03 (-0.24 to 0.30)	

-1   -.5   0   .5   1   1.5

Favours comparison treatment   **Favours manual treatment**

Figure 2.5a: Pooled effect size of manual therapy for non-specific low back pain. From Kent et al.[27]

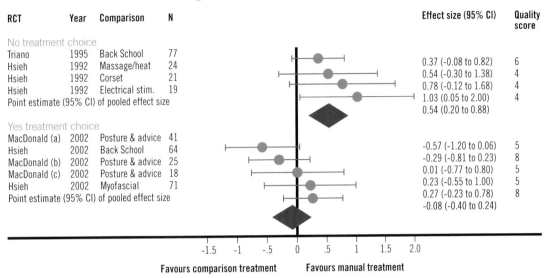

Figure 2.5b: Pooled effect size of manual therapy for activity limitation in non-specific low back pain. From Kent et al.[27]

treatment selection does not improve outcomes in randomized clinical trials of manual therapy for non-specific LBP.

In their conclusion, Kent et al[27] argued that non-specific LBP is heterogeneous and tailoring treatment to subgroups of patients with non-specific LBP should lead to improved patient outcomes. The fact that this was not yet systematically observable could be because of limitations in the design of previous clinical trials, or because tailoring manual therapy treatment to subgroups of patients with non-specific LBP may have minimal effect on pain and activity limitation.[27] They suggested that future research focus on selecting patients for manual therapy clinical trials with a clinical profile that might indicate a likelihood of responding to the manual therapy.[27]

2.6: Clinical Prediction Rule for Manipulation of the Lumbar Spine

Some studies and clinical experience suggest that at least *some* patients with non-specific LBP respond preferentially to spinal TJM treatment interventions. The question has been, how do we identify these patients? Knowing ahead of time which patients are more likely to respond favorably to TJM was the impetus for developing a clinical prediction rule for this. Clinical prediction rules are simply tools in the decision-making process that can improve diagnostic accuracy or predict an outcome. They are combinations of clinical findings that have statistically demonstrated meaningful predictability in determining a selected condition or prognosis of a patient who has been provided a specific treatment or intervention.[28] There are several examples of useful clinical prediction rules in the medical literature including the accuracy of diagnosing ankle fractures,[29] when to order cervical spine radiographs,[30] and diagnosis of cervical radiculopathy.[31]

Flynn et al[32] developed a clinical prediction rule for classifying patients with LBP who demonstrate short-term improvement with TJM. They gathered a sample of the relevant clinical population (patients with LBP) and performed diagnostic tests (everything that might be predictive of success) on all patients in the study. They then performed the reference standard (TJM protocol and a dichotomized clinical outcome) on all patients. Seventy-one patients with LBP were screened for inclusion and exclusion criteria and, once accepted into the study, underwent an exhaustive subjective history and physical examination. Then, regardless of the findings, all patients underwent a standardized supine lumbopelvic TJM technique and were given range of motion exercises. They returned two days later and, if their Oswestry Disability Index had improved by at least 50 percent from their baseline score, they were deemed a 'success.' If they did not improve by at least 50 percent, they were given a repeat of the TJM intervention and range of motion exercises, and asked to return another two days later to determine if they had 'succeeded' or not.[32]

Thirty-two (45%) patients improved dramatically and were classified as a 'success.' A comparison of the 'success' and 'non-success' groups found that the 'success' group had a mean (SD) 73% (16) improvement in their Oswestry Disability Index compared to the 'non-success' group with a mean (SD) 15% (18) improvement.[32] Individual items from the subjective history and physical examination were then tested for their univariate association with the reference standard (success) using independent samples t-tests for continuous variables and χ^2 tests for categorical variables.[32] The items (variables) were then distilled down to a total of 11 potential predictor variables and entered into a logistic regression analysis. Five variables were retained in the final prediction model: duration of symptoms < 16 days; at least one hip with > 35° of internal rotation; hypomobility with lumbar spring testing; Fear-Avoidance Belief Questionnaire Work-Subscale score < 19; and no symptoms distal to the knee.[32] The pre-test probability of experiencing dramatic success (at least 50 percent reduction in Oswestry score) was 45 percent. When patients had at least four out of the five clinical predictors, the positive likelihood ratio was 24.38 (95 percent CI = 4.63 – 139.41) which raised the post-test probability of success to 95 percent (Table 2.6a) and (Table 2.6b).

Based on the use of this newly derived clinical prediction rule, clinicians could assess for the presence of the five predictor variables in their patient, and if at least four were present, could reason that there was a very high (95 percent) probability that they would experience dramatic success with TJM to their lumbar spine.

Table 2.6a: Accuracy statistics with 95 percent confidence intervals for individual variables for predicting success.

Number of Predictor Variables Present	Sensitivity	Specificity	Positive Likelihood Ratio	Probability of Success* (%)
5	0.19 (0.09, 0.35)	1.00 (0.91, 1.00)	∞ (2.02, ∞)	–
4+	0.63 (0.45, 0.77)	0.97 (0.87, 1.00)	24.38 (4.63, 139.41)	95
3+	0.94 (0.80, 0.98)	0.64 (0.48, 0.77)	2.61 (1.78, 4.15)	68
2+	1.00 (0.89, 1.00)	0.15 (0.07, 0.30)	1.18 (1.09, 1.42)	49
1+	1.00 (0.89, 1.00)	0.03 (0.01, 0.13)	1.03 (1.01, 1.15)	46

The probability of success can be calculated using the positive likelihood ratio and assumes a pretest probability of success of 45 percent. Adapted from Flynn et al.[32]

Table 2.6b: Number of subjects in the success and non-success groups at each level of the clinical prediction rule. Adapted from Flynn et al.[32]

Variables in the Clinical Prediction Rule	Number of Predictor Variables Present	Number of Subjects in Success Group	Number of Subjects in Non-success Group
• Symptom duration < 16 days	5	6	0
• No symptoms distal to the knee	4	14	1
• FABQ work subscale score < 19	3	10	13
• Hip internal rotation > 35°	2	2	19
• Hypomobility in lumbar spine	1	0	5
	0	0	1

Childs et al[33] completed a multi-center randomized controlled clinical trial to validate the newly derived clinical prediction rule for TJM of the lumbar spine in patients with LBP. They recruited 131 consecutive patients with LBP and randomly assigned them to receive TJM plus exercise or exercise alone for five sessions over four weeks. Assessment of each patient's status on the clinical prediction rule was not determined until they had completed participation in the study. Subsequently, there was the creation of four groups for statistical analysis: 23 patients who were positive on the rule and received TJM; 47 patients who were negative on the rule and received TJM; 24 patients who were positive on the rule and did not receive TJM; and 37 patients who were negative on the rule and did not receive TJM.[33] While all groups demonstrated improvement in disability (Oswestry) over time, treatment effects were greatest for the subgroup of patients who were positive on the rule and received TJM (Figure 2.6c). Furthermore, health care utilization (medications, seeking continued treatment, and missed time at work)

among that subgroup was decreased at six months.[33] Based on the established pre-test probability of success with TJM of 45 percent, a patient who was positive on the rule (four out of five predictors) and received TJM had a 92 percent post-test probability of a successful outcome (50 percent reduction in Oswestry score).[33] Finally, the associated number needed to treat for benefit at four weeks was 1.9 (95 percent CI = 1.4–3.5) which means that only two patients who are positive on the rule would need to be treated with TJM to prevent one patient from failing to achieve success.

It is important to note that in both the derivation[32] and validation[33] studies on the clinical prediction rule, the interventions of interest (TJM) were not left to the discretion of participating therapists, and the same supine TJM technique was provided to all patients in the first study[32] and all patients in the TJM plus exercise group in the second study.[33] Cleland et al[34] completed a randomized clinical trial to see if using alternative TJM techniques would affect outcomes in patients

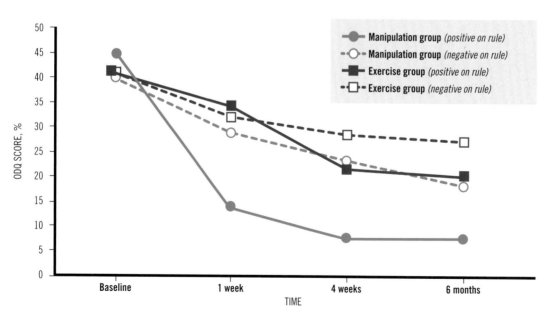

Figure 2.6c: Oswestry Disability Index scores over time for all four groups with manipulation group (positive on rule) having significantly lower scores (less disability) at all follow-up time points. Adapted from Childs et al.[33]

with LBP who satisfied the clinical prediction rule. In that study, 112 patients with LBP who met at least four out of five on the clinical prediction rule were randomized to receive the original supine TJM technique; an alternative side-lying TJM technique; or a prone non-thrust mobilization technique.[34] All patients received five treatment sessions over a four-week period, and only the first two sessions were different between groups. They found a significant group by time interaction for the Oswestry Disability Index (p < 0.001) and pain (p = 0.001).[34] There were no significant differences between the supine and side-lying TJM groups at any time point; however, significant differences existed at each time point between the thrust and non-thrust groups[34] (Figure 2.6d). Disability scores were significantly lower (better) for the thrust versus the non-thrust groups.[34]

The results reported by Cleland et al[34] suggested that it did not matter which TJM technique was provided to patients with LBP who met the clinical prediction rule. However,

it did have to be a TJM technique. Hancock et al[35] conducted a secondary analysis of their randomized controlled trial of manipulation and diclofenac for acute LBP[5] to determine if patients who met the clinical prediction rule had better outcomes (faster recovery) when they received manipulation. They reported that the clinical prediction rule performed no better than chance in identifying patients with acute, non-specific LBP most likely to respond to spinal manipulative therapy.[35] However, in their studies they used a different disability score (Roland-Morris instead of Oswestry).[35] Perhaps more crucially, their participating therapists were able to choose treatment interventions and TJM was only provided in five percent of all treatment sessions to those patients who were assigned to the manipulation group.[5,35]

There has been much debate about the value, or otherwise, of clinical prediction rules in the treatment of musculoskeletal pain. We will discuss this further and offer some thoughts on the best way forward in the chapter on clinical reasoning.

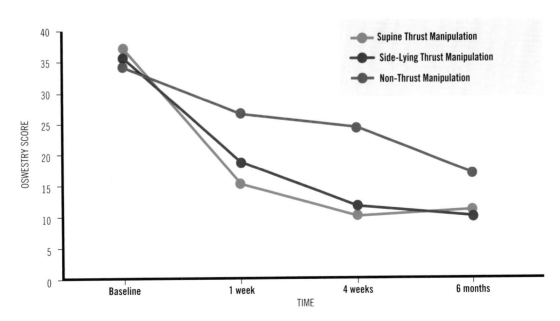

Figure 2.6d: Estimated marginal means for the Oswestry Disability Index scores at each data collection period for all three treatment groups. Adapted from Cleland et al.[34]

2.7: Evidence for the Effectiveness of Thoracic Spine Manipulation

There is surprisingly little research conducted on non-specific thoracic spine pain. Heneghan and Rushton[36] have called the thoracic spine the 'Cinderella' region of the spine, a reference to the lesser research focus compared to the cervical and lumbar regions. A recent randomized clinical trial of thoracic spine manipulation for non-specific thoracic spine pain was published in 2016 by Crothers et al.[37] The authors randomly allocated 143 people with non-specific thoracic pain to one of three groups: spinal manipulative therapy, Graston technique (which is a form of instrument-assisted soft tissue mobilization), or a placebo (de-tuned ultrasound). They found no statistically significant between-group differences in pain or disability at one week, one, three, and six months.[37] They did report significant main effects of time ($p < 0.01$) indicating improvements in pain and disability from baseline for all participants regardless of intervention.[37] It is worth noting that according to the baseline data, all participants had mean symptom duration of 9.2 years, so it is very likely these study participants had chronic pain problems that were no longer associated with thoracic spine tissues. Furthermore, while the manipulation was described as "a series of high velocity low amplitude chiropractic manual adjustments" to the thoracic spine, the thrust direction was at the discretion of the treating clinician.[37]

Southerst et al[38] completed a systematic review to critically appraise and synthesize available evidence on the effectiveness of non-invasive interventions (excluding pharmacological treatments) for musculoskeletal thoracic pain. After screening 6,988 articles, they were left with only two studies to critically appraise. One compared manipulation by a physiotherapist (described as high-velocity thrust between T3 and T8) to acupuncture and to a placebo (de-activated interferential therapy). The other compared a multi-modal program of care provided by a chiropractor (including high-velocity thrust to the cervical and/or thoracic spines) to a single 15-minute consultation for education from a chiropractor. The authors reported statistically significant but clinically non-important short-term reductions in pain favoring manipulation, with no differences between acupuncture and placebo.[38] There was a similar statistically significant but clinically non-important short-term reduction in pain favoring multi-modal care over education.[38] The findings led them to conclude that manipulation was not effective for acute musculoskeletal thoracic spine or chest wall pain.

Much of the available research on thoracic spine manipulation appears to focus on its effects in patients with neck pain, shoulder pain or musculoskeletal dysfunctions other than in the thoracic spine itself. A systematic review and meta-analysis of thrust joint manipulation to the thoracic spine for the management of musculoskeletal dysfunction found 13 randomized clinical trials.[39] However, three of the studies examined thoracic spine manipulation for shoulder pain and dysfunction, nine studies examined it for neck pain, and the final one looked at its effects on lower trapezius muscle strength in asymptomatic subjects. Much of this interest in the use of thoracic spine manipulation in the management of upper quadrant presentations is thought to be linked to the theory of regional interdependence. The thoracic spine is therefore considered as a silent contributor to clinical presentations where pain is felt elsewhere, and not actually in the thorax. We will discuss the evidence for thoracic spine manipulation in patients with neck pain in the next section of this chapter.

2.8: Evidence for the Effectiveness of Cervical Spine Manipulation

Although it has been argued that TJM of the cervical spine "does not work" for neck pain[40], a number of studies have demonstrated that, when combined with exercises, TJM is effective in improving patient outcomes related to neck pain[41-43] and cervicogenic headaches.[44,45] Furthermore, recent systematic reviews also suggest that TJM of the cervical spine is an effective strategy in the management of neck pain[46-48] and cervicogenic headaches.[49-51]

Despite the emergence of evidence in support of the use of cervical spine TJM in patients with neck pain, one recent study suggests that it may not be more beneficial than the mobilization techniques that do not include a high-velocity low-amplitude thrust.[52] Hurwitz and colleagues[52] randomly assigned 336 patients with neck pain to receive either cervical spine manipulation or mobilization, with or without heat, and with or without electrical stimulation. The authors reported that the groups experienced similar outcomes regardless of group assignment, and concluded that mobilization is as effective as manipulation in the management of patients with mechanical neck pain. The results and conclusions drawn from this study need to be interpreted with caution because the study included subjects with varying levels of acuity. Approximately 26 percent had acute neck pain (less than three weeks), 20 percent had sub-acute neck pain (three weeks to three months) and the remaining 54 percent had chronic neck pain (greater than three months).[52] No attempt was made to classify the patients into sub-groupings or sub-classifications of neck pain as proposed by Childs et al[53], and the heterogeneous nature of the patients with neck pain may have significantly affected their results. With such heterogeneity of the subject

population, it is possible that this study failed to show a positive effect for cervical spine TJM because it may have included fewer patients with prognostic factors favoring TJM over non-thrust mobilization.

In contrast to the Hurwitz and colleagues[52] study, a randomized clinical trial by Cassidy et al[54] compared the immediate effects of cervical spine TJM versus mobilization in 100 patients suffering from unilateral neck pain with referral into the trapezius muscle. Fifty-two subjects received a single rotational TJM and 48 subjects received mobilization. Immediate outcome measures were cervical range of motion in three planes and pain intensity rated on the 101-point numerical rating scale. The results showed that both treatments increased range of motion, but cervical spine TJM had a significantly greater effect on reducing pain intensity. While 85 percent of the manipulated patients and 69 percent of the mobilized patients reported pain improvement immediately after treatment, the decrease in pain intensity was more than 1.5 times greater in the manipulated group ($p = 0.05$). They concluded that a single cervical spine TJM was more effective than mobilization in decreasing pain in patients with mechanical neck pain.[54] An analysis of the subjects in the study revealed that 16 had neck pain for less than one week, 34 had pain for between one week and six months while the remaining 50 had pain for more than six months. Therefore, despite the favorable results for cervical spine TJM over mobilization, no attempt was made to classify the patients into sub-groupings or sub-classifications of neck pain as proposed by Childs et al.[53] The degree of the effects of thrust versus non-thrust treatment interventions may have been different with stratification.

Nilsson et al[55] reported on a randomized clinical trial in which 53 subjects suffering from frequent headaches who fulfilled the International Headache Society criteria for cervicogenic headache were randomized to receive cervical spine TJM two times per week for three weeks, or low-level laser in the upper cervical region and deep friction massage (including trigger points) in the lower cervical and upper thoracic region two times a week for three weeks. Outcome measures were analgesic use per day, headache intensity per episode and number of headache hours per day as registered in a headache diary all subjects kept for the five-week intervention. The authors reported significant differences between the groups in all outcome measures in favor of the cervical spine TJM group, and concluded that cervical spine TJM has a significant positive effect in cases of cervicogenic headache. Although the soft tissue techniques used in this study were not graded passive joint mobilizations, it could be argued that the deep friction techniques which included a focus on trigger points may have been somewhat similar to non-thrust mobilization for the cervical spine. A significant strength of this study was that subject selection followed strict inclusion criteria which included the presence of headache five days per month for at least three months, and therefore, some degree of sub-grouping was achieved as all subjects could be classified as having chronic symptoms.

In an earlier study, Nilsson et al[56] examined the effect of cervical spine TJM on passive cervical range of motion. Thirty-nine subjects with headache who objectively demonstrated decreased cervical range of motion were randomized to receive cervical spine TJM two times a week for three weeks (20 subjects) or low-level laser in the upper cervical region and deep friction massage (including trigger points)

in the lower cervical and upper thoracic region twice a week for three weeks (19 subjects). Both groups demonstrated increased passive cervical range of motion during the trial period. However, there were no statistically significant differences between the groups one week after the completion of the treatment. Unfortunately, the study failed to provide information on the subjects other than the fact that they had a mean age of 39 years and demonstrated objectively decreased cervical range of motion in at least one direction. There was no attempt to subgroup the patients according to length or duration of symptoms.

A recent study by Mansilla-Ferragut et al[57] was able to show that the application of an atlantoaxial cervical spine TJM resulted in an increase in active mouth opening and pressure pain threshold over the trigeminal nerve distribution area (sphenoid bone) in women with mechanical neck pain. Thirty-seven women, mean age 35 ± 8 years, with mechanical neck pain were randomly assigned to an experimental group that received atlantoaxial cervical spine TJM and a control group that received a manual contact placebo intervention. Outcomes collected were assessed pre-treatment and five minutes post-treatment by an assessor blinded to the treatment allocation. This included active mouth opening and pressure pain threshold over both sides of the sphenoid bone. Results demonstrated a significant difference between the two groups, with the experimental group showing greater improvement for both measures.[57] The authors had strict inclusion and exclusion criteria for their subject pool, and, of interest, subjects had to have bilateral symptoms that had been present for at least six months. Furthermore, no adverse effects were reported by any participant in the study after the cervical spine TJM procedure.[57]

The benefits of TJM relative to mobilization of the cervical spine need to be weighed against the potential risks. As we will further discuss in the next chapter, the risk of serious complications such as vertebrobasilar artery dissection has been estimated to be extremely low (between five and 10 in 10 million; 0.00005 percent – 0.0001 percent).[58] Many pre-manipulative screening procedures have been proposed to predict patients who may be at risk for serious injury from cervical spine TJM, with much of the attention focused on the vertebral artery.[59-63] Unfortunately, there appears to be little evidence to support these decision-making schemes in their ability to accurately identify these patients[64,65] The lack of evidence for pre-manipulative screening has caused some authors to suggest that identifying patients at risk is virtually impossible[66,67] and others[19,68] to recommend that mobilization may be a safer alternative to TJM. However, serious adverse events have also occurred following mobilization and evidence suggests that TJM may have some value above and beyond that achieved by mobilization or other soft tissue techniques alone.[54,55]

In a recent study, van der Velde et al[69] attempted to identify the best treatment for non-specific neck pain and compared standard non-steroidal anti-inflammatory drugs (NSAIDs), Cox-2 NSAIDs, exercise, mobilization and TJM in a decision-analytic Markov model. Assuming equal effectiveness, they conducted a baseline analysis using risk of harm only and found no significant differences across treatments.[69] Their findings suggested that cervical spine TJM in the management of non-specific neck pain

had equal effectiveness and equal risk of harm when compared to NSAIDs, exercise and mobilization. Interestingly, their target population was defined as persons with neck pain of at least two weeks duration[69] and therefore their model included a heterogeneous sampling of patients with neck pain. It would be interesting to repeat the analysis using subjects with neck pain of less than four weeks' duration.

In their analysis of risks of stroke with cervical spine TJM, van der Velde et al[69] used estimates from two studies[70,71] that reported a positive association between chiropractic visits and posterior circulation (vertebrobasilar) stroke in persons aged < 45 years and a negative association in persons aged ≥ 45 years. The assumption that a chiropractic visit was a reasonable proxy for cervical spine TJM was based on a study that reported 80.8 percent of patients visiting a chiropractor receive cervical spine TJM.[72] However, the study by Cassidy et al[71] found that the incidence of vertebrobasilar artery stroke following a chiropractic visit was no different to the incidence of vertebrobasilar artery stroke following a visit to the primary care physician. They concluded that the increased risk of vertebrobasilar artery stroke associated with chiropractic and primary care physician visits was likely due to patients with headache and neck pain from vertebral artery dissection seeking care *before* their stroke. Another study examined vertebrobasilar artery stroke in two Canadian provinces[73] and found that the increase in vertebrobasilar stroke in Saskatchewan and Ontario in 2000 was not associated with any increase in the rate of chiropractic utilization.

To avoid even the small inherent risks associated with cervical spine TJM, it has been suggested that thoracic spine manipulation interventions may be effective in patients with neck pain.[74] The effectiveness of TJM directed to the thoracic spine in the management of symptoms associated with thoracic pain has been well documented in the literature.[75-79] Recent studies have also demonstrated that thoracic spine TJM in a subgroup of patients with neck pain is effective.[74,80-83]

In a randomized controlled clinical trial, Cleland et al[83] investigated the effectiveness of thoracic spine TJM in a group of patients with mechanical neck pain. Patients admitted to the study completed a baseline historical and physical examination followed by a self-report measure of pain using the visual analog scale. Patients were randomly assigned to receive either a thoracic spine TJM technique or a placebo manipulation technique. A second clinician, blinded to treatment group assignment, would then ask the patient to report their perceived level of neck pain intensity on the visual analog scale within five minutes of completing the treatment.

Thirty-six patients, mean age equal to 36 (SD = 9.8) (27 female), were randomized to receive thoracic spine TJM (n = 19) or a placebo manipulation technique (n = 17). No differences in key demographic variables or levels of pain and disability were noted between the groups at baseline (p > 0.05). A repeated measures ANOVA demonstrated a significant Intervention by Time interaction (p < 0.001) (Figure 2.9a), suggesting that patients receiving thoracic spine TJM experienced immediate improvements in pain compared to patients in the placebo group.

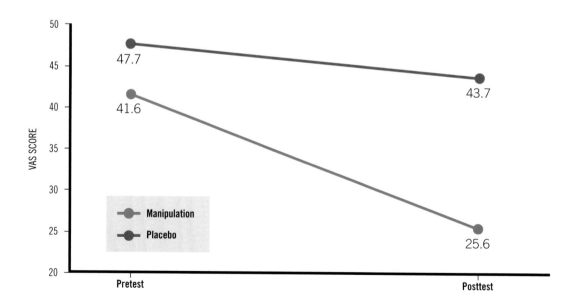

Figure 2.9a: Change in visual analog pain score by group over time. Adapted from Cleland et al.[83]

The authors reported the change in pain in the group receiving thoracic spine TJM was 15.5mm (SD = 7.7) (95 percent CI: 11.8, 19.2), compared to a change in the group receiving placebo manipulation of 4.2mm (SD = 4.6) (95 percent CI: 1.9, 6.6).[83] The results of the study suggested that thoracic spine TJM in patients with a primary complaint of neck pain results in immediate improvements in their neck pain. An analysis of the symptom duration for subjects in both groups, although similar (12.2 weeks, SD = 3.5 manipulation group; and 13.2 weeks, SD = 4.2 placebo manipulation group) indicates that there would have been subjects with acute neck pain (less than four weeks), sub-acute neck pain (four to 12 weeks) and chronic neck pain (more than 12 weeks). No subgrouping or classification of the patients was attempted.

In a follow-up study, Cleland et al[74] developed a clinical prediction to determine *a priori* which patients with neck pain would be more likely to respond favorably to a program of thoracic spine TJM and range of motion exercises. Seventy-eight patients with a primary complaint of neck pain completed a series of self-report measures, and then received a detailed standardized history and physical examination which consisted of a variety of tests and measures commonly used to assess and classify patients with neck pain. Regardless of the history and physical examination findings, all subjects were administered a standardized treatment program consisting of three thoracic spine TJM techniques and a general cervical mobility exercise ("Three-Finger" range of motion exercise). The thoracic TJM techniques included a seated distraction manipulation (known by most clinicians as the 'bear hug' technique); an upper thoracic/cervicothoracic junction supine posterior-anterior thrust technique; and a middle thoracic supine posterior-anterior thrust technique. Depending upon their response to treatment, all subjects were classified as having experienced a successful outcome or not, based on the patient-reported Global Rating of Change Scale (GROC).

Sensitivity, specificity, and positive and negative likelihood ratios were calculated for all variables that were potentially predictive of success on the GROC. Univariate analyses and step-wise logistic regression were used to determine the most parsimonious set of variables for prediction of treatment success. Of the 78 subjects included in the data analysis, 42 reported a successful outcome (54 percent success rate) and the authors were able to derive a clinical prediction rule with six variables (symptom duration < 30 days; no symptoms distal to the shoulder; looking up does not aggravate symptom; Fear Avoidance Beliefs Questionnaire Physical Activity subscale score ≤ 11; decreased upper thoracic spine kyphosis (T3-T5); and cervical extension ROM < 30°). If four of the six predictor variables (+LR = 12) were present, the chance of the subject experiencing a successful outcome improved from 54 percent to 93 percent. Of interest was the fact that duration of symptoms was one of the strongest predictors (+LR = 6.4).[74] This finding was comparable to the clinical prediction rule for LBP, where duration of symptoms < 16 days was also the strongest predictor (+LR = 4.39)[32], and supports studies which have identified that patients who seek care sooner after onset of musculoskeletal conditions have a better prognosis than those who seek care later.[84-90]

The clinical prediction rule derived by Cleland et al[74] was based upon the use of a regional interdependence approach in treating patients with neck pain which is gaining support both clinically and in published reports.[91-95] Treating the thoracic spine in these patients has demonstrated benefits and involves arguably less risk, but may not completely address a patient's presenting symptoms and mobility impairments. It has been our experience that adding cervical spine TJM to a comprehensive management package improves clinical outcomes. We decided to conduct a randomized clinical trial to determine if any differences in outcome would exist when treating patients with neck pain who met the criteria for the clinical prediction rule using cervical spine TJM as opposed to thoracic spine TJM.[96] Twenty-four consecutive patients presenting to physical therapy clinics in the Las Vegas area with a primary complaint of neck pain who met four out of six of the CPR criteria for thoracic spine TJM were randomly assigned to one of two treatment groups. A thoracic group received thoracic spine TJM and cervical range of motion exercises for the first two sessions followed by a standardized exercise program for an additional three sessions. A cervical group received cervical spine TJM and the same cervical range of motion exercises for the first two sessions and received the identical exercises as the thoracic group for their final three sessions. Outcome measures collected at one week, four weeks, and six months from start of treatment included Neck Disability Index (NDI), Numeric Pain Rating Scale (NPRS), and Fear Avoidance Beliefs Questionnaire. All patients also completed a Global Rating of Change Scale (GROC) after the first treatment, after one week, after four weeks, and after six months.

Results from our study demonstrated that patients with neck pain who received cervical spine TJM and exercises demonstrated greater improvements in NDI ($p \leq 0.001$) (Figure 2.9b) and NPRS ($p \leq 0.003$) (Figure 2.9c) at all follow-up time periods.[96] There was also a statistically significant improvement in the FABQ Physical Activity subscale at all follow-ups for the cervical group ($p \leq 0.004$)[96] (Table 2.9d).

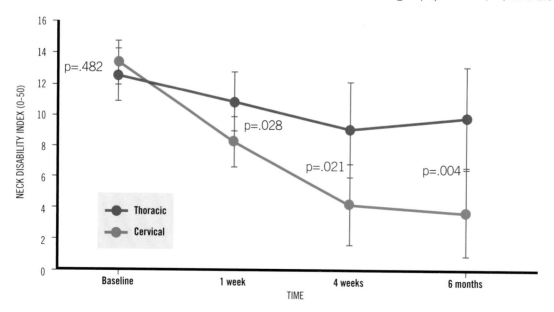

Figure 2.9b: Mean Neck Disability Index Score with 95 percent CI over the course of the trial for the cervical and thoracic manipulation groups. Adapted from Puentedura et al.[96]

Furthermore, we determined absolute risk reduction (ARR) and number needed to treat (NNT) by deeming an outcome as an overall success if the following occurred: NDI score improvement that met or exceeded minimal detectable change (MDC) and minimal clinically important difference (MCID) (7 scale points out of 50); NPRS score improvement that met or exceeded MDC and MCID (2.1 scale points), and a GROC score of at least a +5. If a patient did not meet all three of the aforementioned criteria, then the outcome was deemed unsuccessful.[96]

Ten out of 14 patients in the cervical group achieved improvements in the NDI that met or exceeded the MDC and MCID from baseline to four weeks and baseline to six months whereas only one patient in the thoracic group met or exceeded the MDC and MCID at either follow-up point.[96] The cervical group also experienced more rapid and greater pain relief than the thoracic group. Twelve out of 14 patients in the cervical group achieved

improvements in the NPRS that met or exceeded the MDC and MCID and all patients achieved GROC equal to or greater than +5 within one week.[96] In contrast, only three out of the 10 patients in the thoracic group achieved improvement in the NPRS that met or exceeded the MDC and MCID, and only two out of 10 reported a GROC score equal to or greater than +5 within one week.[96]

The ARR ratio for an unsuccessful outcome from baseline to week one (i.e., those not meeting all three of the success criteria at the end of treatment) was 57.1 percent (95 percent CI: 29.2 percent to 85.1 percent).[96] The associated NNT was found to be 1.8 (95 percent CI: 1.2 to 3.4) in favor of the cervical TJM group.[96] The ARR ratio for the outcome at four weeks was 61.4 percent (95 percent CI: 31.3 percent to 91.5 percent).[96] The NNT was 1.6 (95 percent CI: 1.1 to 3.2), which was also in favor of the cervical TJM group.[96] The ARR and NNT for the outcome at six months were the same as the four-week ARR and NNT.

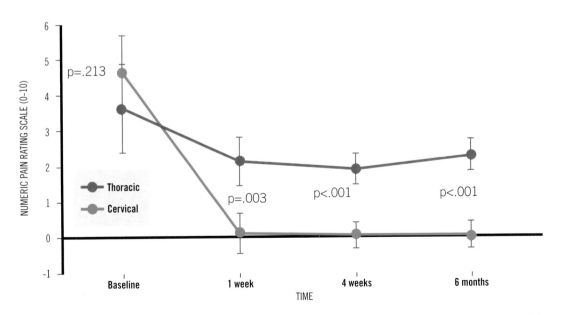

Figure 2.9c: Mean numeric pain rating scale score with 95 percent CI for the intent-to-treat analysis over the course of the trial for the cervical and thoracic manipulation groups. Adapted from Puentedura et al.[96]

Table 2.9d: Outcomes for both groups at each follow-up period. Adapted from Puentedura et al.[96]

Outcome/Group	Baseline	1 Week	4 Weeks	6 months
NDI (0 – 50)				
Thoracic	12.6 ±1.9 (10.9, 14.3)	10.9 ±2.0 (9.0, 12.8)	9.1 ±3.7; 6.0, 12.2)	9.9 ±3.9 (6.6, 13.2)
Cervical	13.4 ±2.9 (11.9, 14.8)	8.3 ±3.4 (6.7, 9.9)	4.2 ±5.4 (1.6, 6.8)	3.7 ±5.7 (0.9, 6.5)
NPRS (0 – 10)				
Thoracic	3.6 ±1.4 (2.4, 4.9)	2.1 ±1.6 (1.5, 2.8)	1.9 ±1.0 (1.5, 2.3)	2.3 ±1.1 (1.9, 2.8)
Cervical	4.6 ±2.2 (3.6, 5.7)	0.1 ±0.2 (-0.5, 0.7)	0.05 ±0.1 (-0.3, 0.4)	0.05 ±0.1 (-0.3, 0.4)
FABQPA (0 – 24)				
Thoracic	8.0 ±4.0 (5.4, 10.6)	5.5 ±3.6 (3.3, 7.7)	4.0 ±2.7 (1.9, 6.1)	5.2 ±3.0 (3.0, 7.4)
Cervical	9.7 ±4.1 (7.5, 12.0)	2.9 ±3.3 (1.0, 4.8)	2.4 ±3.4 (0.7, 4.2)	2.1 ±3.5 (0.3, 4.0)

* Data are mean ± SD, 95 percent CI
(Abbreviations: SD = standard deviation; NDI = neck disability index; NPRS = numeric pain rating scale; FABQPA = Fear avoidance beliefs questionnaire – physical activity subscale)

We also found that patients receiving cervical spine TJM demonstrated fewer transient side-effects compared to the patients receiving thoracic spine TJM for their neck pain.[96] The results of our study provided some encouragement for another project on identifying variables in patients with neck pain that would predict a favorable outcome with cervical spine TJM.

Cleland et al[97] completed a recent validation study for their clinical prediction rule for neck pain responsive to thoracic TJM. In a randomized controlled clinical trial, they randomly assigned 140 patients with a primary report of neck pain to one of two groups. An exercise-only group received five sessions of stretching and strengthening exercises and a manipulation plus exercise group received two sessions of thoracic TJM and cervical range of motion exercises followed by a final three sessions of the same stretching and strengthening exercises as the exercise-only group. They collected data on disability and pain at baseline, one week, four weeks, and six months, and conducted a linear mixed model with repeated measures to assess the primary aim (treatment group * time * status on the clinical prediction rule). They found no three-way interaction for either disability (p = 0.79) (Figure 2.9e) or pain (p = 0.22) (Figure 2.9f).[97] These findings suggested that outcomes over time were not dependent upon the combination of a patient's treatment group and status on the clinical prediction rule.

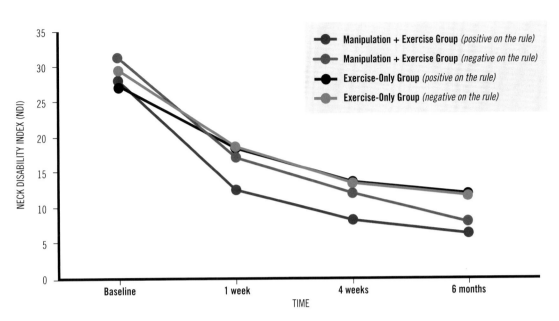

Figure 2.9e: Mean Scores for Neck Disability Index (NDI) by group assignment over time. Adapted from Cleland et al.[97]

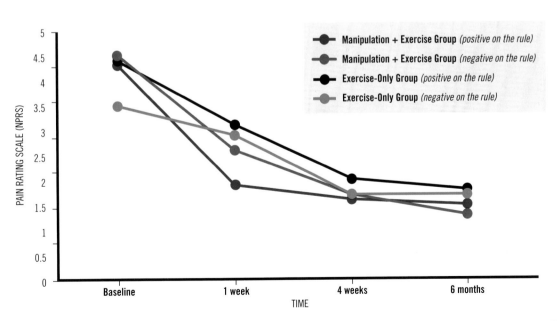

Figure 2.9f: Mean scores for Numeric Pain Rating Scale (NPRS) by group assignment over time. Adapted from Cleland et al.[97]

However, a two-way (group * time) interaction existed for both disability and pain.[97] Pairwise comparisons of disability (NDI) showed that significant differences existed at each follow-up period in favor of the manipulation plus exercise group when compared to the exercise-only group. Patients who received thoracic TJM as part of their treatment also reported lower pain scores at the one-week follow-up period (Figure 2.9g).

The results did not support the validity of the clinical prediction rule. However, the authors demonstrated that patients with mechanical neck pain who received thoracic TJM and exercise exhibited significantly greater improvements in pain and disability compared with patients who received exercise only.

The failure of this validation study meant that the clinical prediction rule did not help identify patients with mechanical neck pain who would demonstrate greater improvements when provided with thoracic TJM in addition to exercise. Instead, the findings suggested that patients with neck pain (and no contraindications for thoracic TJM) who were given a combination of thoracic TJM and exercise had statistically and clinically significantly greater improvements in pain and disability compared to exercise alone.[97] Clinicians reading the research report might conclude (rightly or wrongly) that *all* patients with mechanical neck pain and no contraindications to TJM should receive thoracic TJM regardless of their clinical presentation (i.e. status on a clinical prediction rule).

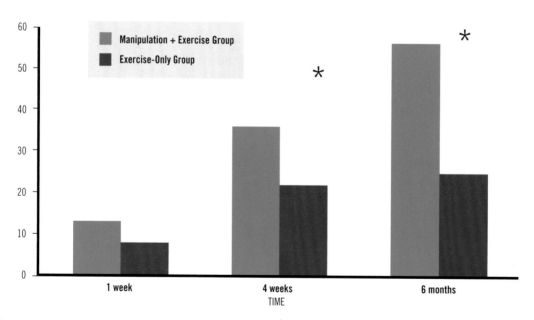

Figure 2.9g: Success rates across time for each group, with success defined as scoring +5 or greater on the Global Rating Of Change Scale (GROC). Adapted from Cleland et al.[97]

*=significant difference (p<.05)

2.10: Clinical Prediction Rule for Manipulation of the Cervical Spine

Based on the findings of our randomized controlled trial of cervical versus thoracic spine TJM in patients with neck pain,[96] we conducted a single cohort study to develop a clinical prediction rule for patients with neck pain who were likely to benefit from cervical spine TJM.[98] In that study, 82 patients with a primary complaint of neck pain were screened for strict inclusion and exclusion criteria, then completed a series of self-report measures, and received a detailed and exhaustive standardized history and physical examination. Regardless of the history and physical examination findings, all subjects were administered a standardized treatment program consisting of an upslope or rotation cervical spine TJM technique to each side of their neck and a general cervical mobility exercise ("Three-Finger" range of motion exercise). All subjects were classified as having experienced a successful outcome or not, based on the patient-reported Global Rating of Change Scale (GROC).

Sensitivity, specificity, and positive and negative likelihood ratios were calculated for all variables that were potentially predictive of success on the GROC. Univariate analyses and step-wise logistic regression were used to determine the most parsimonious set of variables for prediction of treatment success.

Of the 82 subjects included in the data analysis, 32 (39 percent) reported dramatic improvement on the GROC and were classified as a 'success' and a comparison of the 'success' and 'non-success' groups found that the 'success' group had a mean 59 percent improvement in their Neck Disability Index compared to the 'non-success' group with a mean 39 percent improvement.[98] We were able to derive a clinical prediction rule with four variables (symptom duration < 38 days; positive expectation that manipulation would help; difference in cervical rotation range of motion to either side at least 10°; and pain with spring testing the middle cervical spine [C3-C5]).

If a patient with neck pain presented with three of the four predictor variables, the positive likelihood ratio was 13.5 (95 percent CI = 4.5 – 41.1) which raised the post-test probability of success to 90 percent (Table 2.10a) and (Table 2.10b). Based on the use of this newly derived clinical prediction rule, clinicians could assess for the presence of the four predictor variables in their patient, and if at least three were present, could reason that there was a very high (90 percent) probability that they would experience dramatic success with TJM to their cervical spine.

Table 2.10a: Accuracy statistics with 95 percent confidence intervals for individual variables for predicting success.

Number of Predictor Variables Present	Sensitivity	Specificity	Positive Likelihood Ratio	Probability of Success* (%)
4	0.50	1.00	Infinite	100%
3+	0.81	0.94	13.5 (4.5 – 41.1)	90%
2+	1.00	0.70	3.3 (2.1 – 4.9)	68%
1+	1.00	0.16	1.2 (1.0 – 1.4)	43%

* The probability of success can be calculated using the positive likelihood ratio and assumes a pretest probability of success of 39 percent. Adapted from Puentedura et al.[98]

Table 2.10b: Number of subjects in the success and non-success groups at each level of the clinical prediction rule. Adapted from Puentedura et al.[98]

Variables in the Clinical Prediction Rule

- Symptom duration < 38 days
- Positive expectation that manipulation will help
- Difference in cervical rotation range of motion to either side at least 10°
- Pain with spring testing middle cervical spine

Number of Predictor Variables Present	Number of Subjects in Success Group	Number of Subjects in Non-success Group
4	16	0
3	10	3
2	6	12
1	0	27
0	0	8

We also compared the treatment effect for cervical spine TJM in all 82 patients in the study versus the effect size in only those patients who met the newly derived clinical prediction rule.[98] For the Neck Disability Index, the entire study sample improved by 7.1 points (out of 50) from baseline. Those who were positive on the rule (n = 29) improved by 8.7 points whereas those who were negative on the rule (n = 53) improved by 6.2 points. The difference between groups was 2.5 points and this was significant (p = 0.021).[98] The effect size, calculated as the mean NDI change score for those negative on the rule minus the mean NDI change score for those positive on the rule divided by the pooled standard deviations, was 0.55 (Cohen's d) which is considered to be a medium effect size.

For the NPRS, the entire study sample improved by 2.1 points (out of 10) from baseline. Those who were positive on the rule (29) improved by 3.5 points whereas those who were negative on the rule (53) improved by 1.3 points. The difference between groups was 2.1 points and this was significant (p < 0.001).[98] The effect size, calculated as the mean NPRS change score for those negative on the rule minus the mean NPRS change score for those positive on the rule divided by the pooled standard deviations, was 1.37 (Cohen's d) which is considered to be a large effect size.

We are currently conducting a randomized clinical trial to attempt to validate the newly derived clinical prediction rule. It is anticipated that up to 200 patients with a primary complaint of neck pain will be required for this study, as the percentage of patients who meet the clinical prediction rule is only about 30 percent. This means that once they are randomized to either a cervical spine TJM plus exercise group or exercise-only group and complete the study, only 60 will likely be positive on the rule whereas 140 will likely be negative on the rule. Because the projected 60 who might be positive on the rule will be divided into a TJM or an exercise group, this will likely leave us with about 30 in each group for analysis.

As previously mentioned, there has been much debate about the value, or otherwise, of clinical prediction rules in the treatment of musculoskeletal pain, and we will discuss this further and offer some thoughts on the best way forward in the chapter on clinical reasoning.

2.11: Key Points from Chapter 2

- The evidence for the effectiveness of TJM to the spine is only moderate at best, but this may well be because research designs fail to account for heterogeneity of patients with low back pain, and variability in the provision of TJM.

- Evidence of effectiveness for TJM appears stronger when sub-grouping provides more homogeneous samples of patients with LBP.

- There is evidence that study outcomes are improved when participating therapists provide experimental interventions prescriptively rather than them having a choice in what interventions to provide (pragmatic designs).

- A clinical prediction rule has been developed and validated for a sub-group of patients with LBP who respond dramatically to TJM.

- The clinical prediction rule that was developed for patients with neck pain who would respond to thoracic spine TJM was not successfully validated. Instead, it was found that all patients with neck pain who have no contraindications for TJM are likely to benefit from thoracic spine TJM compared to exercise alone.

- A clinical prediction rule for patients with neck pain who are likely to benefit from cervical spine TJM has been developed, but the validation of this rule has not been completed.

Chapter 2 References

1. APTA. Evidence-Based Practice & Research. 2017; http://www.apta.org/EvidenceResearch/. Accessed April 2017.

2. Hoffman T, Bennett S, Del Mar C. *Evidence-Based Practice: Across the Health Professions.* 2nd ed. Chatswood, NSW: Elsevier; 2013.

3. Smith GC, Pell JP. Parachute use to prevent death and major trauma related to gravitational challenge: systematic review of randomised controlled trials. *BMJ.* 2003;327(7429):1459-1461.

4. Rothberg S, Friedman BW. Complementary therapies in addition to medication for patients with nonchronic, nonradicular low back pain: a systematic review. *Am J Emerg Med.* 2017; 35(1):55-61.

5. Hancock MJ, Maher CG, Latimer J, et al. Assessment of diclofenac or spinal manipulative therapy, or both, in addition to recommended first-line treatment for acute low back pain: a randomised controlled trial. *Lancet.* 2007;370(9599):1638-1643.

6. Juni P, Battaglia M, Nuesch E, et al. A randomised controlled trial of spinal manipulative therapy in acute low back pain. *Ann Rheum Dis.* 2009;68(9):1420-1427.

7. Ruddock JK, Sallis H, Ness A, Perry RE. Spinal Manipulation Vs Sham Manipulation for Nonspecific Low Back Pain: A Systematic Review and Meta-analysis. *J Chiropr Med.* 2016;15(3):165-183.

8. Bronfort G, Haas M, Evans R, Leininger B, Triano J. Effectiveness of manual therapies: the UK evidence report. *Chiropr Osteopat.* 2010;18:3.

9. Licciardone JC, Brimhall AK, King LN. Osteopathic manipulative treatment for low back pain: a systematic review and meta-analysis of randomized controlled trials. *BMC Musculoskelet Disord.* 2005;6:43.

10. Rubinstein SM, van Middelkoop M, Assendelft WJ, de Boer MR, van Tulder MW. Spinal manipulative therapy for chronic low-back pain: an update of a Cochrane review. *Spine (Phila Pa 1976).* 2011;36(13):E825-846.

11. Rubinstein SM, Terwee CB, Assendelft WJ, de Boer MR, van Tulder MW. Spinal manipulative therapy for acute low-back pain. *Cochrane Database Syst Rev.* 2012(9):CD008880.

12. von Heymann WJ, Schloemer P, Timm J, Muehlbauer B. Spinal high-velocity low amplitude manipulation in acute nonspecific low back pain: a double-blinded randomized controlled trial in comparison with diclofenac and placebo. *Spine (Phila Pa 1976).* 2013;38(7):540-548.

13. Senna MK, Machaly SA. Does maintained spinal manipulation therapy for chronic nonspecific low back pain result in better long-term outcome? *Spine (Phila Pa 1976).* 2011;36(18):1427-1437.

14. Merepeza A. Effects of spinal manipulation versus therapeutic exercise on adults with chronic low back pain: a literature review. *J Can Chiropr Assoc.* 2014;58(4):456-466.

15. Cecchi F, Negrini S, Pasquini G, et al. Predictors of functional outcome in patients with chronic low back pain undergoing back school, individual physiotherapy or spinal manipulation. *Eur J Phys Rehabil Med.* 2012;48(3):371-378.

16. Ferreira ML, Ferreira PH, Latimer J, et al. Comparison of general exercise, motor control exercise and spinal manipulative therapy for chronic low back pain: A randomized trial. *Pain.* 2007;131(1-2):31-37.

17. Goldby LJ, Moore AP, Doust J, Trew ME. A randomized controlled trial investigating the efficiency of musculoskeletal physiotherapy on chronic low back disorder. *Spine (Phila Pa 1976).* 2006;31(10):1083-1093.

18. Paige NM, Miake-Lye IM, Booth MS, et al. Association of Spinal Manipulative Therapy With Clinical Benefit and Harm for Acute Low Back Pain: Systematic Review and Meta-analysis. *JAMA.* 2017;317(14):1451-1460.

19. Childs JD, Piva SR, Fritz JM. Responsiveness of the numeric pain rating scale in patients with low back pain. *Spine (Phila Pa 1976).* 2005;30(11):1331-1334.

20. Rice ME, Harris GT. Comparing effect sizes in follow-up studies: ROC Area, Cohen's d, and r. *Law Hum Behav.* 2005;29(5):615-620.

21. Team UBT. United Kingdom back pain exercise and manipulation (UK BEAM) randomised trial: effectiveness of physical treatments for back pain in primary care. *BMJ.* 2004;329(7479):1377.

22. Ostelo RW, de Vet HC. Clinically important outcomes in low back pain. *Best Pract Res Clin Rheumatol.* 2005;19(4):593-607.

23. Harvey E, Burton AK, Moffett JK, Breen A, team UBt. Spinal manipulation for low-back pain: a treatment package agreed to by the UK chiropractic, osteopathy and physiotherapy professional associations. *Man Ther.* 2003;8(1):46-51.

24. Underwood MR, Harding G, Klaber Moffett J, team UBt. Patient perceptions of physical therapy within a trial for back pain treatments (UK BEAM) [ISRCTN32683578]. *Rheumatology (Oxford).* 2006;45(6):751-756.

25. Hurwitz EL, Morgenstern H, Kominski GF, Yu F, Chiang LM. A randomized trial of chiropractic and medical care for patients with low back pain: eighteen-month follow-up outcomes from the UCLA low back pain study. *Spine (Phila Pa 1976).* 2006;31(6):611-621; discussion 622.

26. Cecchi F, Molino-Lova R, Chiti M, et al. Spinal manipulation compared with back school and with individually delivered physiotherapy for the treatment of chronic low back pain: a randomized trial with one-year follow-up. *Clin Rehabil*. 2010;24(1):26-36.

27. Kent P, Marks D, Pearson W, Keating J. Does clinician treatment choice improve the outcomes of manual therapy for nonspecific low back pain? A metaanalysis. *J Manipulative Physiol Ther*. 2005;28(5):312-322.

28. Beattie P, Nelson R. Clinical prediction rules: what are they and what do they tell us? *Aust J Physiother*. 2006;52(3):157-163.

29. Stiell IG, Greenberg GH, McKnight RD, Nair RC, McDowell I, Worthington JR. A study to develop clinical decision rules for the use of radiography in acute ankle injuries. *Ann Emerg Med*. 1992;21(4):384-390.

30. Stiell IG, Wells GA, Vandemheen KL, et al. The Canadian C-spine rule for radiography in alert and stable trauma patients. *JAMA*. 2001;286(15):1841-1848.

31. Wainner RS, Fritz JM, Irrgang JJ, Boninger ML, Delitto A, Allison S. Reliability and diagnostic accuracy of the clinical examination and patient self-report measures for cervical radiculopathy. *Spine (Phila Pa 1976)*. 2003;28(1):52-62.

32. Flynn T, Fritz J, Whitman J, et al. A clinical prediction rule for classifying patients with low back pain who demonstrate short-term improvement with spinal manipulation. *Spine (Phila Pa 1976)*. 2002;27(24):2835-2843.

33. Childs JD, Fritz JM, Flynn TW, et al. A clinical prediction rule to identify patients with low back pain most likely to benefit from spinal manipulation: a validation study. *Ann Intern Med*. 2004;141(12):920-928.

34. Cleland JA, Fritz JM, Kulig K, et al. Comparison of the effectiveness of three manual physical therapy techniques in a subgroup of patients with low back pain who satisfy a clinical prediction rule: a randomized clinical trial. *Spine (Phila Pa 1976)*. 2009;34(25):2720-2729.

35. Hancock MJ, Maher CG, Latimer J, Herbert RD, McAuley JH. Independent evaluation of a clinical prediction rule for spinal manipulative therapy: a randomised controlled trial. *Eur Spine J*. 2008;17(7):936-943.

36. Heneghan NR, Rushton A. Understanding why the thoracic region is the 'Cinderella' region of the spine. *Man Ther*. 2016;21:274-276.

37. Crothers AL, French SD, Hebert JJ, Walker BF. Spinal manipulative therapy, Graston technique(R) and placebo for non-specific thoracic spine pain: a randomised controlled trial. *Chiropr Man Therap*. 2016;24:16.

38. Southerst D, Marchand AA, Cote P, et al. The effectiveness of noninvasive interventions for musculoskeletal thoracic spine and chest wall pain: a systematic review by the Ontario Protocol for Traffic Injury Management (OPTIMa) collaboration. *J Manipulative Physiol Ther*. 2015;38(7):521-531.

39. Walser RF, Meserve BB, Boucher TR. The effectiveness of thoracic spine manipulation for the management of musculoskeletal conditions: a systematic review and meta-analysis of randomized clinical trials. *J Man Manip Ther*. 2009;17(4):237-246.

40. Bogduk N. Spinal manipulation for neck pain does not work. *J Pain*. 2003;4(8):427-428; discussion 429-430.

41. Evans R, Bronfort G, Nelson B, Goldsmith CH. Two-year follow-up of a randomized clinical trial of spinal manipulation and two types of exercise for patients with chronic neck pain. *Spine*. 2002;27(21):2383-2389.

42. Bronfort G, Evans R, Nelson B, Aker PD, Goldsmith CH, Vernon H. A randomized clinical trial of exercise and spinal manipulation for patients with chronic neck pain. *Spine*. 2001;26(7):788-797; discussion 798-789.

43. Wilson S. Spinal manipulation and exercise for chronic neck pain: are they more effective when delivered alone or in combination? *Aust J Physiother*. 2001;47(4):300.

44. Jull G, Trott P, Potter H, et al. A randomized controlled trial of exercise and manipulative therapy for cervicogenic headache. *Spine*. 2002;27(17):1835-1843; discussion 1843.

45. Gross AR, Kay TM, Kennedy C, et al. Clinical practice guideline on the use of manipulation or mobilization in the treatment of adults with mechanical neck disorders. *Man Ther*. 2002;7(4):193-205.

46. Bronfort G, Haas M, Evans RL, Bouter LM. Efficacy of spinal manipulation and mobilization for low back pain and neck pain: a systematic review and best evidence synthesis. *Spine J*. 2004;4(3):335-356.

47. Gross AR, Hoving JL, Haines TA, et al. A Cochrane review of manipulation and mobilization for mechanical neck disorders. *Spine*. 2004;29(14):1541-1548.

48. Gross AR, Hoving JL, Haines TA, et al. Manipulation and mobilisation for mechanical neck disorders. *Cochrane Database Syst Rev*. 2004(1):CD004249.

49. Biondi DM. Physical treatments for headache: a structured review. *Headache*. 2005;45(6):738-746.

50. Fernandez-de-Las-Penas C, Alonso-Blanco C, Cuadrado ML, Pareja JA. Spinal manipulative therapy in the management of cervicogenic headache. *Headache*. 2005;45(9):1260-1263.

51. Fernandez-de-Las-Penas C, Alonso-Blanco C, Cuadrado ML, Miangolarra JC, Barriga FJ, Pareja JA. Are manual therapies effective in reducing pain from tension-type headache?: a systematic review. *Clin J Pain*. 2006;22(3):278-285.

52. Hurwitz EL, Morgenstern H, Harber P, Kominski GF, Yu F, Adams AH. A randomized trial of chiropractic manipulation and mobilization for patients with neck pain: clinical outcomes from the UCLA neck-pain study. *Am J Public Health*. 2002;92(10):1634-1641.

53. Childs JD, Fritz JM, Piva SR, Whitman JM. Proposal of a classification system for patients with neck pain. *JOSPT*. 2004;34(11):686-696; discussion 697-700.

54. Cassidy JD, Lopes AA, Yong-Hing K. The immediate effect of manipulation versus mobilization on pain and range of motion in the cervical spine: a randomized controlled trial. *J Manipulative Physiol Ther*. 1992;15(9):570-575.

55. Nilsson N, Christensen HW, Hartvigsen J. The effect of spinal manipulation in the treatment of cervicogenic headache. *J Manipulative Physiol Ther*. 1997;20(5):326-330.

56. Nilsson N, Christensen HW, Hartvigsen J. Lasting changes in passive range motion after spinal manipulation: a randomized, blind, controlled trial. *J Manipulative Physiol Ther*. 1996;19(3):165-168.

57. Mansilla-Ferragut P, Fernandez-de-Las Penas C, Alburquerque-Sendin F, Cleland JA, Bosca-Gandia JJ. Immediate effects of atlanto-occipital joint manipulation on active mouth opening and pressure pain sensitivity in women with mechanical neck pain. *J Manipulative Physiol Ther*. 2009;32(2):101-106.

58. Hurwitz EL, Aker PD, Adams AH, Meeker WC, Shekelle PG. Manipulation and mobilization of the cervical spine. A systematic review of the literature. *Spine*. 1996;21(15):1746-1759; discussion 1759-1760.

59. Refshauge KM, Parry S, Shirley D, Larsen D, Rivett DA, Boland R. Professional responsibility in relation to cervical spine manipulation. *Aust J Physiother*. 2002;48(3):171-179; discussion 180-175.

60. Grant R. Vertebral artery testing - the Australian Physiotherapy Association Protocol after 6 years. *Man Ther*. 1996;1(3):149-153.

61. Rivett DA. The pre-manipulative vertebral artery testing protocol: a brief review. *New Zealand Journal of Physiotherapy* 1995;1:9 - 12.

62. Barker S, Kesson M, Ashmore J, Turner G, Conway J, Stevens D. Professional issue. Guidance for pre-manipulative testing of the cervical spine. *Man Ther*. 2000;5(1):37-40.

63. Licht PB, Christensen HW, Hoilund-Carlsen PF. Is there a role for premanipulative testing before cervical manipulation? *J Manipulative Physiol Ther*. 2000;23(3):175-179.

64. Bolton PS, Stick PE, Lord RS. Failure of clinical tests to predict cerebral ischemia before neck manipulation. *J Manipulative Physiol Ther*. 1989;12(4):304-307.

65. Cote P, Kreitz BG, Cassidy JD, Thiel H. The validity of the extension-rotation test as a clinical screening procedure before neck manipulation: a secondary analysis. *J Manipulative Physiol Ther*. 1996;19(3):159-164.

66. Haldeman S, Kohlbeck FJ, McGregor M. Risk factors and precipitating neck movements causing vertebrobasilar artery dissection after cervical trauma and spinal manipulation. *Spine*. 1999;24(8): 785-794.

67. Haldeman S, Kohlbeck FJ, McGregor M. Unpredictability of cerebrovascular ischemia associated with cervical spine manipulation therapy: a review of sixty-four cases after cervical spine manipulation. *Spine*. 2002;27(1):49-55.

68. Jull G. Use of high and low velocity cervical manipulative therapy procedures by Australian manipulative physiotherapists. *Aust J Physiother*. 2002;48(3):189-193.

69. van der Velde G, Hogg-Johnson S, Bayoumi AM, et al. Identifying the best treatment among common nonsurgical neck pain treatments: a decision analysis. *Spine*. 2008;33(4 Suppl):S184-191.

70. Rothwell DM, Bondy SJ, Williams JI. Chiropractic manipulation and stroke: a population-based case-control study. *Stroke*. 2001;32(5):1054-1060.

71. Cassidy JD, Boyle E, Cote P, et al. Risk of vertebrobasilar stroke and chiropractic care: results of a population-based case-control and case-crossover study. *Spine*. 2008;33(4 Suppl):S176-183.

72. Hurwitz EL, Coulter ID, Adams AH, Genovese BJ, Shekelle PG. Use of chiropractic services from 1985 through 1991 in the United States and Canada. *Am J Public Health*. 1998;88(5):771-776.

73. Boyle E, Cote P, Grier AR, Cassidy JD. Examining vertebrobasilar artery stroke in two Canadian provinces. *Spine*. 2008;33(4 Suppl):S170-175.

74. Cleland JA, Childs JD, Fritz JM, Whitman JM, Eberhart SL. Development of a clinical prediction rule for guiding treatment of a subgroup of patients with neck pain: use of thoracic spine manipulation, exercise, and patient education. *Phys Ther*. 2007;87(1):9-23.

75. Menck JY, Requejo SM, Kulig K. Thoracic spine dysfunction in upper extremity complex regional pain syndrome type I. *JOSPT*. 2000;30(7):401-409.

76. Chok B, Wong WP. Treatment of unilateral upper thoracic vertebral pain using an eclectic approach. *Physiother Res Int*. 2000;5(2):129-133.

77. Schiller L. Effectiveness of spinal manipulative therapy in the treatment of mechanical thoracic spine pain: a pilot randomized clinical trial. *J Manipulative Physiol Ther*. 2001;24(6):394-401.

78. Pho C, Godges J. Management of whiplash-associated disorder addressing thoracic and cervical spine impairments: a case report. *JOSPT*. 2004;34(9):511-519; discussion 520-513.

79. Austin GP, Benesky WT. Thoracic pain in a collegiate runner. *Man Ther*. 2002;7(3):168-172.

80. Gonzalez-Iglesias J, Fernandez-de-las-Penas C, Cleland JA, Gutierrez-Vega Mdel R. Thoracic spine manipulation for the management of patients with neck pain: a randomized clinical trial. *JOSPT*. 2009;39(1):20-27.

81. Gonzalez-Iglesias J, Fernandez-de-Las-Penas C, Cleland JA, Alburquerque-Sendin F, Palomeque-Del-Cerro L, Mendez-Sanchez R. Inclusion of thoracic spine thrust manipulation into an electro-therapy/thermal program for the management of patients with acute mechanical neck pain: A randomized clinical trial. *Man Ther*. 2008.

82. Cleland JA, Glynn P, Whitman JM, Eberhart SL, MacDonald C, Childs JD. Short-term effects of thrust versus nonthrust mobilization/manipulation directed at the thoracic spine in patients with neck pain: a randomized clinical trial. *Phys Ther*. 2007;87(4):431-440.

83. Cleland JA, Childs JD, McRae M, Palmer JA, Stowell T. Immediate effects of thoracic manipulation in patients with neck pain: a randomized clinical trial. *Man Ther*. 2005;10(2):127-135.

84. Wand BM, Bird C, McAuley JH, Dore CJ, MacDowell M, De Souza LH. Early intervention for the management of acute low back pain: a single-blind randomized controlled trial of biopsychosocial education, manual therapy, and exercise. *Spine*. 2004;29(21):2350-2356.

85. Zigenfus GC, Yin J, Giang GM, Fogarty WT. Effectiveness of early physical therapy in the treatment of acute low back musculoskeletal disorders. *J Occup Environ Med*. 2000;42(1):35-39.

86. Ehrmann-Feldman D, Rossignol M, Abenhaim L, Gobeille D. Physician referral to physical therapy in a cohort of workers compensated for low back pain. *Phys Ther*. 1996;76(2):150-156; discussion 156-157.

87. Linton SJ, Hellsing AL, Andersson D. A controlled study of the effects of an early intervention on acute musculoskeletal pain problems. *Pain*. 1993;54(3):353-359.

88. Slater MA, Weickgenant AL, Greenberg MA, et al. Preventing progression to chronicity in first onset, subacute low back pain: an exploratory study. *Arch Phys Med Rehabil*. 2009;90(4):545-552.

89. Lebec MT, Jogodka CE. The physical therapist as a musculoskeletal specialist in the emergency department. *JOSPT*. 2009;39(3):221-229.

90. Curtis C, d'Hemecourt P. Diagnosis and management of back pain in adolescents. *Adolesc Med State Art Rev*. 2007;18(1):140-164, x.

91. Bialosky JE, Bishop MD, George SZ. Regional interdependence: a musculoskeletal examination model whose time has come. *JOSPT*. 2008;38(3):159-160; author reply 160.

92. Strunce JB, Walker MJ, Boyles RE, Young BA. The immediate effects of thoracic spine and rib manipulation on subjects with primary complaints of shoulder pain. *J Man Manip Ther*. 2009;17(4):230-236.

93. Wainner RS, Whitman JM, Cleland JA, Flynn TW. Regional interdependence: a musculoskeletal examination model whose time has come. *JOSPT*. 2007;37(11):658-660.

94. Vicenzino B, Collins D, Wright A. The initial effects of a cervical spine manipulative physiotherapy treatment on the pain and dysfunction of lateral epicondylalgia. *Pain*. 1996;68(1):69-74.

95. Vicenzino B, Collins D, Benson H, Wright A. An investigation of the interrelationship between manipulative therapy-induced hypoalgesia and sympathoexcitation. *J Manipulative Physiol Ther*. 1998;21(7):448-453.

96. Puentedura EJ, Landers MR, Cleland JA, Mintken PE, Huijbregts P, Fernandez-de-Las-Penas C. Thoracic spine thrust manipulation versus cervical spine thrust manipulation in patients with acute neck pain: a randomized clinical trial. *JOSPT*. 2011;41(4):208-220.

97. Cleland JA, Mintken PE, Carpenter K, et al. Examination of a clinical prediction rule to identify patients with neck pain likely to benefit from thoracic spine thrust manipulation and a general cervical range of motion exercise: multi-center randomized clinical trial. *Phys Ther*. 2010;90(9):1239-1250.

98. Puentedura EJ, Cleland JA, Landers MR, Mintken PE, Louw A, Fernandez-de-Las-Penas C. Development of a clinical prediction rule to identify patients with neck pain likely to benefit from thrust joint manipulation to the cervical spine. *J Orthop Sports Phys Ther*. 2012;42(7):577-592.

Chapter 3

Safety of Thrust Joint Manipulation

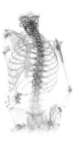

3.1: Chapter Objectives

Safety with thrust joint manipulation (TJM) is a significant concern for all therapists, and in this chapter, we present a detailed discussion of the safety concerns. We include the two systematic reviews of case reports of adverse events following TJM to the cervical and thoracic spines that we authored, as well as a third systematic review of case reports of adverse events following TJM to the lumbar spine. Results from that research make the case for sound clinical reasoning in the determination of appropriateness of using TJM techniques. We also discuss the results of a recent survey study of physical therapists in the US concerning their thoughts about TJM.

3.2: Primum Non Nocere (First, Do No Harm)

Primum non nocere is a Latin phrase that means "first, do no harm" and it is considered a part of the Hippocratic Oath which has historically been taken by physicians entering the profession. While therapists are not required to take the oath as they embark upon entry to the profession, the maxim of "Do no Harm" is firmly embedded into the lexicon. With any treatment technique or intervention, clinicians must weigh the risks and benefits for the patient before them, and choose appropriately. Why is it that TJM is perceived by many therapists as posing far greater risks than most other interventions they may use in clinical practice? The answer to that question may be found by conducting a Google search using the words "neck manipulation dangerous," which will result in a torrent of articles and stories on tragedies that have been attributed to TJM in the cervical spine.

A *Washington Post* article by Susan Berger in January 2014[1] entitled "How safe are the vigorous neck manipulations done by chiropractors?" reported on two women who were harmed by TJM to their cervical spine. One became dizzy and unable to see or move after having a chiropractor work on her neck.

She was rushed to a hospital where a shunt was inserted to relieve pressure caused by swelling in her brain. She had suffered a series of strokes and eight years later was still suffering from constant vertigo. The second woman was a retired lieutenant colonel in the army and reportedly knew she was in trouble seconds after a chiropractor in Oklahoma City manipulated her neck. Because of her years as a combat medic in Kosovo and Somalia, she realized what was happening and yelled, "Stop. I'm having a stroke." More than a decade later, she is reported to be blind in her left eye and having problems with swallowing due to paralysis of one side of her throat.

A more recent story in the news media involves the death of 34-year-old Playboy model Katie May after visiting a chiropractor for her neck pain.[2] In that case, the Los Angeles County coroner attributed the death to the actions of the chiropractor, and ruled the cause of death was vertebral artery dissection. Similar stories can be found for serious adverse events following TJM to the thoracic and lumbar spines. It is therefore not unreasonable for a therapist to be concerned about risks associated with these treatment techniques.

3.3: Risks and Side Effects Associated with Cervical Spine Manipulation

Much attention has been given to the potential risks associated with the administration of TJM to the cervical spine.[3-7] Di Fabio[3] completed a review of previously reported cases in which injuries were attributed to manipulation of the cervical spine. He found 177 published cases of injury reported in 116 articles published between 1925 and 1997.[3] The most frequently reported injuries involved arterial dissection or spasm and lesions of the brain stem. Death occurred in 32 (18 percent) of the cases, and none of the serious irreversible events were attributed to TJM performed by physical therapists.[3] The majority of the adverse events were attributed to TJM performed by chiropractors (Figure 3.3a).

Ernst[9] completed a systematic review of case reports of serious adverse events following TJM to the cervical spine from 1995 – 2001. A total of 42 individual cases were found in which arterial dissection causing stroke occurred in 18 patients.[9] The author concluded that serious adverse events after TJM were continuing to be reported, and further prospective studies were needed to more accurately define the risks associated with TJM to the cervical spine.

In a subsequent systematic review of papers published between January 2001 and June 2006, Ernst[10] sought to further identify the adverse effects of TJM. The review included a total of 32 case reports, four retrospective case series, two prospective case series, three case-control studies and three surveys. Findings were that the most serious problems are vertebral artery dissections due to intimal tearing thought to be due to stretching during rotational TJM. Although symptoms were reported as 'frequently life-threatening,' most of the 32 patients in the case reports made a full recovery and no deaths were reported.[10]

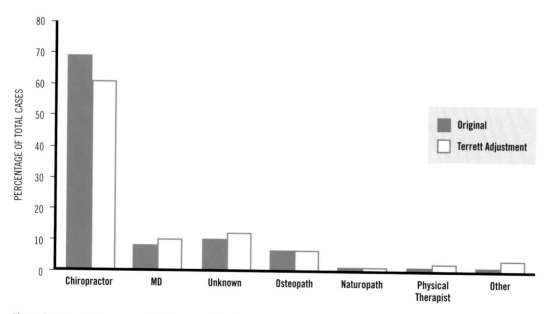

Figure 3.3a: Practitioners reported to have provided Thrust Joint Manipulation (TJM) to the cervical spine that resulted in serious adverse events. For the purpose of comparison, the type of practitioner was adjusted according to findings by Terrett.[8] Adapted from Di Fabio.[3]

Data provided from these three reviews found that TJM, particularly when performed on the upper cervical spine, was associated with mild to moderate adverse effects. Furthermore, this could also result in serious complications such as vertebral artery dissection followed by stroke.[3,9,10] However, the reviews by Di Fabio[3] and Ernst[9,10] were largely descriptive in nature providing data on the age, sex and diagnosis of the patients involved as well as the type of clinician providing the TJM; the type of TJM technique; the nature of the adverse events; and the clinical outcome. The only conclusion therapists could draw after reading these reviews was that TJM to the cervical spine was a risk, and perhaps they should not be doing it. There was little to no guidance on how to minimize risks and side effects associated with TJM to the cervical spine.

Because of this, we conducted a systematic narrative review on the safety of TJM to the cervical spine to determine if adverse events were preventable and if TJM was being performed appropriately.[11] Case reports published in peer-reviewed journals involving adverse events following TJM to the cervical spine were found by searching PubMed (1950-2010) and the Cumulative Index to Nursing and Allied Health (CINHAL, 1982-2010). We defined an adverse event as the sequelae following a TJM that are medium to long-term in duration, with moderate to severe symptoms, and of a nature that was serious, distressing, and unacceptable to the patient and required further treatment.[12] Identified case reports were analyzed in a fashion similar to previously conducted reviews[3,9,10] for information on gender; age; who performed the TJM and why; presence of contraindications; the number of TJM interventions performed; initial symptoms

experienced after the TJM; as well as type of adverse event that resulted. Based on the information gathered, TJMs were categorized as appropriate or inappropriate, and adverse events were categorized as preventable, unpreventable or unknown. The appropriateness of cases was dichotomized based upon the patient's presenting condition. A case was determined to be appropriate if TJM was used for an indicated condition such as neck pain, neck stiffness, headache, or cervical radiculopathy; and inappropriate when TJM to the cervical spine was performed for reasons that are not indicative to cervical disorders, such as LBP, otitis media, asthma, non-radicular shoulder pain or maintenance therapy.

Preventability was based on the presence of factors that increase a patient's risk for injury. Cases were classified as preventable when contraindications to TJM should have otherwise stopped the care provider from performing TJM and unpreventable when the patient appeared to be clear of any contraindications to TJM either in the current and/or past history. Therefore, a TJM to the cervical spine could have been performed for appropriate reasons, but if the clinician performed the TJM in the presence of contraindications, the adverse event was classified as preventable. Cases were also classified as preventable when TJM to the cervical spine was continued for more than five consecutive treatment sessions with either no change in presenting symptoms or worsening of symptoms. An unknown category was created and used whenever a case report did not provide enough information to allow it to be categorized as either preventable or unpreventable.

Chi-square analysis with an alpha level of .05 was used to determine if there was a difference in proportion between the six categories: appropriate/preventable, appropriate/unpreventable, appropriate/unknown, inappropriate/preventable, inappropriate/unpreventable and inappropriate/unknown. Our hypothesis was that there would be an association between TJMs that were performed inappropriately and adverse events that were preventable.

One hundred thirty-four cases, reported in 93 articles, were analyzed for our review and involved 73 males and 61 females. The average age of the patient was 43.8 years (SD = 11.8, Range= 23 to 86 years).[11] Arterial dissection was the most common adverse event reported, being present in 37.3 percent of the cases (n = 50). Other common adverse events included disc herniation (18.7 percent, n = 25), CVA (13.4 percent, n = 18), and vertebral dislocation or fracture (6.7 percent, n = 9).[11] Chiropractors were involved in the majority of the adverse events following TJM to the cervical spine with 69.4 percent (n = 93) of the cases analyzed (Figure 3.3b).

Chi-square analysis showed no significant difference in the proportions between appropriateness of the TJM and preventability of adverse events, p = 0.459. Of the cases analyzed, 19.4 percent (n = 26) of the TJMs were categorized as inappropriate, 44.8 percent (n = 60) of the AE were preventable, and nine percent (n = 12) of these were both deemed inappropriate and preventable (Table 3.3c). There was no significant association between appropriateness of TJM and preventability of adverse events, indicating that TJMs performed inappropriately were not more likely to be classified as preventable. In fact, while 80.6 percent of all reviewed TJMs were performed for appropriate conditions, 44.8 percent of the cases were preventable and apparently not screened for contraindicating signs. Our results suggested that simply determining that a TJM may be indicated is not sufficient to prevent an adverse event.

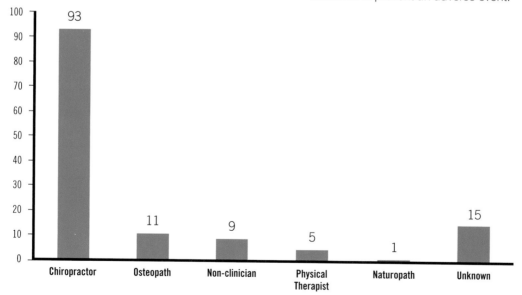

Figure 3.3b: Frequency counts of practitioners performing TJM to the cervical spine in reported cases of serious adverse events. Adapted from Puentedura et al.[11]

Table 3.3c: Distribution of Cases Categorized by Appropriateness and Preventability. Adapted from Puentedura et al.[11]

	Appropriate	Inappropriate	Total
Preventable	48	12	60
	80.0%	20.0%	44.8%
Unpreventable	13	1	14
	92.9%	7.2%	10.4%
Unknown	47	13	60
	78.3%	21.7%	44.8%
Total	108	26	134
	80.6%	19.4%	100.0%

We concluded that from a clinical perspective, a thorough examination to rule out all contraindications to TJM may have the potential to prevent nearly half of all adverse events related to TJM. Of the 74 cases that could be classified as either preventable or unpreventable, 60 (81 percent) were preventable and 14 (19 percent) were unpreventable.

If the 60 cases classified as unknown were to be allocated in the same proportions, then 49 (81 percent of 60) would have been preventable and 11 (19 percent of 60) would have been unpreventable. Therefore, we could speculate that of the 134 total cases, 109 (81.3 percent) were preventable and 25 (18.7

percent) were unpreventable, and there may be potential to prevent over 80 percent of all adverse events related to TJM to the cervical spine (Table 3.3d).

Additionally, 19.4 percent of TJMs reviewed were performed for inappropriate conditions, meaning patients were placed at risk for an adverse event although they were not likely to benefit from the technique.[11] We argue that by performing a thorough examination and using sound clinical reasoning, clinicians may be able to prevent almost all adverse events, further reducing risks associated with TJM and improving patient safety.

Table 3.3d: Distribution of cases categorized by appropriateness and preventability after adjusting for unknown category.

	Appropriate	Inappropriate	Total
Preventable	48	12	109
	80.0%	20.0%	81.3%
Unpreventable	13	1	25
	92.9%	7.2%	18.7%
Total	108	26	134
	80.6%	19.4%	100.0%

Studies have also shown that there are relatively high incidences of side effects with the application of TJM.[13-27] These side effects include local discomfort, headache, tiredness, and radiating discomfort. They are reported to be transient in nature, and lasting no longer than 24 hours. A study by Senstad et al[13] reviewed data from 4,712 treatments on 1,058 new patients by 102 Norwegian chiropractors and found that at least one side effect was reported by 55 percent of the patients sometime during the course of a maximum of six treatments. The most common side effect was local discomfort, which accounted for 53 percent of all reported reactions (Figure 3.3e). Headache, tiredness, radiating discomfort and dizziness accounted for 12 percent, 11 percent, 10 percent and five percent of all reported side effects respectively.

Cagnie et al[17] conducted a survey regarding adverse reactions associated with TJM in Belgium. Fifty-nine manipulative therapists (physiotherapists, osteopaths and chiropractors) participated in the study. They asked 15 consecutive patients who received TJM to the spine as part of their initial treatment to complete a survey on any adverse reactions (side effects) they experienced within 48 hours of their treatment. A total 639 questionnaires were analyzed and adverse reactions varied from headache (20 percent) and stiffness (19 percent) to dizziness (four percent) and nausea (three percent) (Figure 3.3f). The majority of the patients (61 percent) reported that their adverse reactions began within four hours of their treatment, and 64 percent reported resolution of those symptoms within 24 hours. Predictors of experiencing a headache after TJM to the spine included gender, with females more likely to experience side effects (Odds Ratio (OR):1.66; 95 percent CI: 1.01 – 2.75); use of medication (OR: 2.20; 95 percent CI: 1.31 – 3.69); and age (OR: 1.02; 95 percent CI: 1.00 – 1.05).[17]

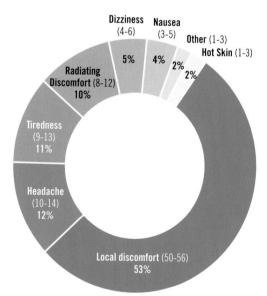

Figure 3.3e: Side Effects of Spinal Manipulation Reported. Adapted from Senstad et al.[13]

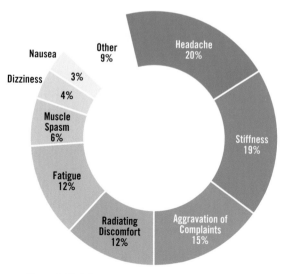

Figure 3.3f: Adverse Reactions to Spinal Manipulation Reported. Adapted from Cagnie et al.[17]

Unfortunately, the authors did not clearly indicate which region of the spine (cervical, thoracic, or lumbar) was associated with what percentage of the overall side effects. In fact, it appears that the clinicians may have applied spinal TJM to two or more regions, as the average number of manipulations per patient was two, with 28.5 percent of the cases receiving three or more manipulations during one session.[17] Of the 930 recorded manipulations, 38.6 percent included the cervical spine, 25.7 percent the thoracic spine, 23.6 percent the lumbar spine and 12.1 percent the sacroiliac joint.[17]

It is extremely difficult to quantify the risk associated with TJM to the cervical spine and various estimates for a serious complication (adverse event) range between five and 10 per 10 million manipulations.[28] Many pre-manipulative screening procedures have been proposed to predict patients who may be at risk for serious injury from TJM, with much of the attention focused on the vertebral artery.[7,29-32] Unfortunately, there appears to be little evidence to support these decision-making schemes in their ability to accurately identify these patients.[33,34] The lack of evidence for pre-manipulative screening has caused some to suggest that identifying patients at risk is virtually impossible[5,35]. This caused others[19,36] to recommend that non-thrust mobilization may be a safer alternative to TJM. However, serious adverse events have also occurred following non-thrust mobilization. Furthermore, evidence suggests that TJM may have some value above and beyond that achieved by non-thrust mobilization or other soft tissue techniques alone.[37,38]

Several studies have attempted to quantify the risk of serious adverse events associated with TJM to the cervical spine. Rothwell et al[39] reviewed hospitalization records to identify vertebrobasilar accidents (VBAs) in Ontario,

Canada, during 1993-1998 and found 582 cases within that five-year period. They age and gender matched each of the 582 cases to controls from the Ontario population with no history of stroke at the event date, then accessed public health insurance billing records to document use of chiropractic services before the event date. They found that for those aged < 45 years, VBA cases were five times more likely than controls to have visited a chiropractor within one week of the VBA (95 percent CI: 1.32 – 43.87).[39] Additionally, for those aged < 45 years, VBA cases were five times as likely to have had at least three chiropractic visits with a cervical diagnosis in the month before the case's VBA date (95 percent CI: 1.34 – 18.57).[39] No significant associations were found for those older than 45 years. Vertebral artery dissections in younger people has been shown to occur spontaneously without any motion, trauma or TJM to the cervical spine,[40] and may have more to do with the health of the patient's vascular system.

Cassidy et al[41] conducted a population-based, case crossover study in Ontario, Canada, where all incidences of carotid artery stroke admitted to hospitals over a nine-year period were identified. Cases served as their own controls and exposure to chiropractic versus primary care physician services were determined from health billing records. They compared 15,523 cases to 60,092 control periods using exposure windows of one, three, seven and 14 days prior to the stroke. Positive associations were found for both chiropractic and primary care physician visits and subsequent stroke in patients less than 45 years of age, but there was no significant difference between chiropractic and primary care physician risk estimates.[41] It was just as likely that patients less than 45 years old suffering a stroke had visited a primary care physician (and, presumably, not had neck manipulation) rather than a chiropractor.

In an earlier study, Cassidy et al[42] investigated associations between chiropractic visits and vertebrobasilar (VBA) stroke and contrasted this with primary care physician visits and VBA stroke. They reported on 818 VBA strokes, and in those aged less than 45 years, cases were about three times more likely to see either a chiropractor or a primary care physician before their stroke than controls.[42] Of greater interest was the finding that, although there was no significant association between chiropractic visits and VBA strokes in those aged over 45 years, there were positive associations between primary care physicians and VBA stroke in all age groups.[42] They reported that practitioner visits billed for headache and neck pain complaints were highly associated with subsequent VBA stroke.[42]

Thomas et al[43] examined the medical records of patients from the Hunter region of New South Wales, Australia aged ≤ 55 years with radiographically confirmed or suspected vertebral or internal carotid artery dissection. They retrospectively compared these patients with matched controls who had suffered stroke from some other cause. From records of 47 dissection patients (27 males, mean age 37.6 years) and 43 stroke controls (22 males, mean age 42.6 years), they found that mild mechanical trauma to the head and neck was significantly associated with craniocervical artery dissection.[43] In fact, using adjusted odds ratios, they reported that dissection patients were 23.51 (95 percent CI = 5.71 – 96.89) times more likely to have sustained minor mechanical head and neck trauma, and they were 12.67 (95 percent CI = 1.43 – 112.0) times more likely to have had manual therapy to their neck. Interestingly, the descriptions of the minor mechanical trauma included heavy lifting, sports activities, turning quickly, and even a wisdom tooth extraction.[43] They concluded that clinicians should be on the lookout for the possibility of arterial dissection in a patient presenting with headache or neck pain and reporting a recent history of even minor head and neck trauma.

In a second study involving the same population in Australia, Thomas et al[44] compared 24 patients with cervical arterial dissection and 21 matched patients with ischemic stroke but not dissection. They found that 17 of the 24 patients with dissections reported a recent history of minor mechanical trauma or neck strain within the last month, and it was more common in those with vertebral artery dissection (nine out of 10) than those with internal carotid artery dissection (eight out of 14).[44] The reported mechanism of trauma or neck strain were broadly classified as either jerky or abrupt head movement, intense or unusual physical effort, and sustained extreme positions of the neck.[44] Overall, patients with arterial dissections were 60 (95% CI = 8.7 - ∞) times more likely to have been exposed to recent minor mechanical trauma or neck strain than those in the comparison ischemic stroke group (p <.001).[44] Only four of the 24 patients had undergone recent chiropractic treatment of their neck in the month prior to their arterial dissection, and although they were 5.2 (95 percent CI = 0.6 - ∞) times more likely to have undergone recent thrust joint manipulation to their cervical spine that those in the comparison group, it was not statistically significant.[44]

Taken together, the above studies suggest that vascular dysfunction leading to strokes in people under the age of 45 years occur just as frequently whether a person has been to a chiropractor (and had TJM to their cervical spine) or not. As clinicians, we should therefore be screening for any possible dysfunction in the cervical arterial system, as symptoms of such vascular dysfunction often present as headaches and neck pain. Kerry and Taylor[45-50] have written extensively on the subject of hemodynamic assessment and screening for cervical arterial dysfunction as an integral part of the evaluation prior to provision of any manual therapy to the cervical spine. Checking blood pressure as part of the manual assessment of someone complaining of headaches and neck pain might seem novel to manual therapists with years of clinical practice, but evidence suggests it should become a routine screening tool in the drive to eliminate serious adverse events associated with any manual therapy to the cervical spine.

3.4: Risks and Side Effects Associated with Thoracic Spine Manipulation

Compared to the cervical and lumbar regions, there appears to be very little in the research literature on the safety of TJM when applied to the thoracic spine, and indeed it appears that many therapists may be more comfortable providing it to this area of the spine as opposed to the cervical and lumbar regions.[51] TJM to the thoracic spine has been recommended in the management of patients with mechanical neck pain (as a less risky alternative to TJM to the cervical spine);[52-55] found to provide short-term success in some individuals with shoulder pain;[56,57] and also reported to be beneficial in the management of temporomandibular disorders when combined with mobilization with movement and dry needling.[58]

While it appears to receive scant attention within the research literature, it is evident that there are risks associated with TJM to the thoracic spine just as there are in the other areas of the spine. We felt that many therapists may have held naïve notions of relative safety when applying TJM to the thoracic spine, so we searched for systematic reviews of serious adverse events on this subject. Finding none, we set out to perform a systematic review and retrospectively analyzed all available documented case reports in the literature describing patients who had experienced severe adverse events after receiving TJM to their thoracic spine.[59] Case reports published in peer-reviewed journals involving adverse events following TJM to the thoracic spine were found by searching all available online databases including PubMed and the Cumulative Index to Nursing and Allied Health (CINHAL) from January 1950 to February 2015.

A total of 10 cases, reported in seven articles, were found and analyzed (Table 3.4a). The cases involved two males and eight females with a mean age of 43.5 years (SD = 18.73, Range = 17 – 71).[59] The most frequent adverse event was injury (mechanical or vascular) to the spinal cord (seven cases). The next most reported AE was pneumothorax and hematothorax (two cases) and cerebrospinal fluid (CSF) leak secondary to dural sleeve injury was reported in the final case.[59] Chiropractors were involved in the majority of injuries following TJM to the thoracic spine with seven of the cases analyzed. An osteopathic physician, physical therapist and a lay person were involved in the remaining three of the cases.

Table 3.4a: The 10 cases of serious adverse events reported in seven published articles.

#	Authors and year	Age (years), sex	Interval to symptom onset	Practitioner	Thoracic level manipulated	Adverse event
1	Ruelle et al., 1999	64, F	2 h	Chiropractor	Lumbar and thoracic spine	Acute epidural hematoma T9-11
2		60, F	Not Known	Chiropractor	Upper thoracic spine	T4-5 collapse; cord compression
3	Oppenheim et al., 2005	56, F	Not Known	Chiropractor	Upper thoracic spine	T4 pathology; epidural tumor
4		71, F	Not Known	Chiropractor	Upper thoracic spine	T4 fracture; lung CA
5		32, M	Not Known	Chiropractor	Middle thoracic spine	Thoracic syrinx, swollen cord
6	Lopez-Gonzalez and Peris-Celda, 2011	45, F	2 h	Chiropractor	Middle thoracic spine	Traumatic T8-T9 disc herniation; complete T6 level paraplegia secondary to spinal cord ischemia
7	Lee et al., 2011	38, F	4 h	Chiropractor	Cervical and upper thoracic spine	Acute epidural hematoma T1-7
8	Struewer et al., 2013	17, M	2 days	Osteopath	Middle thoracic spine	Large left hematothorax
9	Masneri et al., 2007	20, F	24 h	Lay Person	Middle thorax	Right pneumothorax
10	Donovan et al., 2007	32, F	2 weeks	Physical Therapist	Cervical and upper thoracic spine	CSF leak and spontaneous intracranial hypotension from dural sleeve tear C8-T5

All these cases were published by neurosurgery and emergency medicine physicians providing patient care following the AE. They found that there was insufficient information in the case reports to determine if the TJM provided to the thoracic spine was appropriate. They also asked if there were any contraindications or precautions to TJM in the thoracic spine that could have alerted the clinician providing the TJM to increased risks of adverse events and hence prevented them. It is possible that the therapists providing the TJM may have failed to recognize signs of these underlying issues, but equally, it is possible that the patients presented without such signs for the therapists to detect. The inability to recognize such signs may be attributed to the lack of reliable and valid screening tools, as well as poor history taking and insufficient clinical reasoning. However, it is also possible that therapists had no intent to screen for contraindications due to lack of knowledge, poor clinical judgement, or carelessness. Regardless of the evidence, or lack thereof, it is the responsibility of the therapist to perform screening examinations and clearly document their use to reduce legal risk if an adverse event was to occur with TJM to the thoracic spine.

Our review[59] showed that serious adverse events do occur in the thoracic spine. Because the most commonly reported injury was trauma to the spinal cord followed by pneumothorax, it suggests that excessive peak forces may have been applied to the thoracic spine. Such findings should serve as a cautionary note for therapists to thoroughly examine their patients, use sound clinical reasoning, and work on their skills to decrease peak forces associated with TJM to the thoracic spine.

3.5: Risks and Side Effects Associated with Lumbar Spine Manipulation

What are the risks (if any) of TJM to the lumbar spine? This is a valid question to ask, and while most practicing manual therapists might suggest that the risks are so minimal as to be non-existent, the literature suggests that there is some concern about causing harm. Take, for example, an often quoted study on the efficacy of physiotherapy/physical therapy for low back pain (LBP). Frost et al[60] conducted a well-designed pragmatic, multi-center, randomized controlled trial of physiotherapy compared with advice for LBP. They had 286 patients with LBP and randomized them to receive advice only and a back book (n=142) or physiotherapy and a back book (n=144). The outcomes were followed at two, six and 12 months using the Oswestry Disability Index (ODI) as well as the Roland Morris Disability Questionnaire (RMDQ) and SF-36. They reported no significant difference in disease-specific and generic outcomes between the two groups. Furthermore, they concluded that routine physiotherapy seemed to be no more effective than one session of assessment and advice from a therapist.[60] However, a look at what "physiotherapy" was provided to the patients with LBP revealed it was commonly low velocity spinal joint mobilization and specific exercises and TJM was provided in only three percent of the treatments. The question to be asked is why TJM was so rarely utilized when there is strong evidence for its effectiveness in this population? Perhaps the answer might be that therapists are fearful of causing harm. Adams and Sim[14] conducted a postal survey of 300 UK manipulative therapists and had a 50 percent response rate with 129 respondents identifying themselves as providers of TJM.

Anxiety about possible complications and fear of litigation were the primary reasons for therapists to not provide TJM, even in the lumbar spine.[14]

Haldeman and Rubinstein[61] conducted a review of the available literature over a 77-year period from 1911 to 1989 and found only 10 reported cases of cauda equina syndrome (a serious adverse event) in patients undergoing lumbar spine manipulation without anesthesia. They estimated the risk of such an adverse event following TJM to the lumbar spine to be less than one per 10 million manipulations. In a more recent systematic review of cases, Hebert et al[62] looked at serious adverse events and TJM to the low back region. They searched all available databases up to January 2012 and found 41 studies reporting on 77 cases. Adverse events were primarily cauda equina syndrome (38 percent of cases) with the rest involving lumbar disc herniation (30 percent); fracture (9 percent); and other serious adverse events (23 percent). They found that important case details were frequently unreported. This included things such as descriptions of the TJM technique used, details of the presentation of the patient before TJM, and specific details of the adverse event, etc. Therefore, they could not draw any causal inferences between TJM to the lumbar spine and the adverse events identified in their review.[62] What these two studies indicate is that serious adverse events following TJM to the lumbar spine are extremely rare. Indeed, some authors have estimated it to be of the order of less than one case per 100 million manipulations.[63,64]

3.6: Putting the Risks of Spinal Manipulation into Perspective

When considering appropriate interventions for spinal pain and disability, therapists should certainly consider the risks and benefits of available treatment options. How does the risk of TJM compare to the risk associated with other medical interventions for patients with neck or back pain?

A common approach by medical practitioners is to prescribe non-steroidal anti-inflammatory drugs (NSAIDs) and advice to keep active. However, taking NSAIDs is not without risk. Studies have reported that long-term use has an overall incidence of symptomatic or endoscopic gastrointestinal (GI) toxicity of approximately 20 percent, and the incidence of life-threatening GI bleeding or perforation is one percent to three percent.[65] As many as 7,600 deaths and 76,000 hospitalizations annually in the US may be attributable to long-term and unnecessary prescriptions for NSAIDs,[66] and it has been reported that one in 1,000 patients will experience a GI bleed if they take NSAIDs for longer than four weeks.[67]

With respect to the advice to keep active, it should be noted that the risk of sudden death is estimated to be one in 1.5 million episodes of vigorous physical exertion.[68] In another study of complications from therapeutic modalities where 362 total complications were documented, it was found that the use of icepacks (cryotherapy) accounted for 42 percent, electrical stimulation 29 percent, therapeutic heat 22 percent and therapeutic exercise seven percent of complications.[69] If we accept that the risk of a serious complication (cauda equina syndrome) following TJM to the lumbar spine is one in 10 million, then the estimated occurrence per 10,000 administrations would be 0.001. Also, the risk of a serious complication (death, stroke) following TJM to the cervical spine is five to 10 in 10 million, then again, the estimated occurrence per 10,000 administrations would be between 0.005 – 0.010. As the risk of sudden death with exercise is one in 1.5 million, the estimated occurrence per 10,000 episodes would be 0.007. This would be seven times higher than TJM to the lumbar spine. Similarly, the risk of a GI bleed with long-term NSAIDs use is one to three in 100. So the estimated occurrence per 10,000 would be 100 – 300 (Table 3.6a).

Table 3.6a: Comparative analysis of the risks of potential complications from interventions for low back pain.

Procedure	Reported Risk	Est #/10K	Potential Complication
Lumbar Manipulation	1/ 10 Million	0.001	Cauda Equina
Cervical Manipulation	5 – 10/ 10 Million	0.005 – 0.010	Death, Stroke
Exercise	1/ 1.5 Million	0.007	Sudden death
NSAIDs	1 – 3/ 100	100 - 300	GI Bleed

A greater concern with respect to the treatment of neck and low back pain should be the harm caused by failing to provide treatment interventions that could have led to improvement. Failure to improve from neck or low back pain could be viewed as a potential complication associated with the non-use of TJM interventions. Childs et al[70] conducted a secondary analysis to determine if patients who did not receive TJM for their LBP would be at an increased risk for worsening disability compared to patients receiving TJM and exercise. They reported that patients who had exercise without TJM were eight times more likely to experience a worsening in disability (defined as ≥ six point increase in the ODI) than patients who did receive TJM one week after the start of treatment.[70] These patients were also four times more likely to experience worsening at four weeks, and three times more likely at six months.[70] Patients with LBP who have continued symptoms and disability beyond four weeks are at greater risk for chronic disability and work restrictions,[71-73] and they account for a disproportionate number of healthcare dollars and worker's compensation costs.[73,74] Therefore, as the risks associated with harm due to TJM to the lumbar spine are almost negligible, the risk of not offering TJM to patients is real, and a more bold approach seems to be warranted. Gordon Waddell wrote, "Orthodox medicine has a long way to go to reduce the rate of serious complications of most of our investigations and treatments to the order of 1:0.2-1 million." He further stated, "What matters is the balance of effectiveness versus risk, and that is strongly in favor of manipulation."[75]

3.7: Utilization of Spinal Manipulation by US Physical Therapists

A recent survey of physical therapist professional degree programs in the US found that all but one of the 147 responding programs were currently teaching TJM in their curriculum.[76] An interesting finding was that of the spinal regions, the cervical spine received the least amount of emphasis, with 52 out of 147 (35 percent) responding programs not teaching TJM to the cervical spine.[76] This is in contrast to TJM in the lumbar and thoracic regions, which was taught in virtually all responding programs (99 percent and 97 percent respectively).[76] Although an increase from the 47 percent of responding programs that excluded cervical techniques found in an earlier study,[77] it indicated that cervical spine TJM is not taught to the same degree as TJM for other spinal regions. If therapists are not being taught cervical spine TJM in their first professional degree programs, we can only assume that those wishing to learn and safely practice this intervention must be looking to post-professional programs such as manual therapy certification, orthopedic residencies and/or fellowships.

As previously discussed, TJM in the cervical spine remains under-utilized compared to the other regions of the spine, and this fact, combined with the fewer teaching opportunities for it, led us to wonder how TJM to the spine is viewed by therapists currently practicing in the US. Therefore, we completed a survey of physical therapists to determine their utilization of TJM within the three spinal regions, their thoughts about safety and efficacy of TJM to the spinal regions, and any perceived barriers to utilization of TJM.[51] We received completed surveys from 1,000 licensed physical therapists in the US, and had 478 males (48 percent) with a mean age of respondents of 39.7 ± 10.81 years, who had mean years of experience of 13.6 ± 10.62 years in clinical practice.[51] The majority of responding therapists agreed that TJM was safe and effective when applied to the lumbar (90.5 percent) and thoracic (91.1 percent) spines; however, a significantly smaller percentage (68.9 percent) agreed with that for the cervical spine (Figure 3.7a). More therapists agreed they would perform additional medical and physical screening before using TJM in the cervical spine as compared to the lumbar and thoracic spines (Figure 3.7b). Finally, therapists agreed they were less likely to provide and feel comfortable with TJM in the cervical spine compared to the thoracic and lumbar spines (Figures 3.7c and 3.7d).

Thrust Joint Manipulation in the XXX spine is safe and effective for patients in which it is indicated

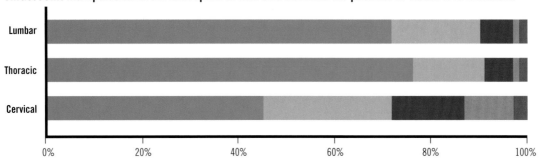

Figure 3.7a: Levels of agreement with the statement "Thrust Joint Manipulation in the XXX spine is safe and effective for patients in which it is indicated."

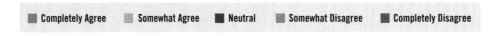

Prior to performing Thrust Joint Manipulation to the XXX spine, I would routinely perform additional medical history screening

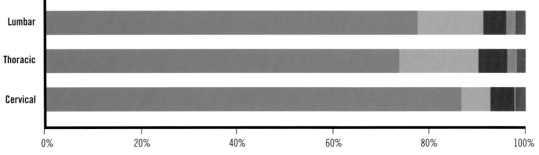

Figure 3.7b: Levels of agreement with the statement "Prior to performing Thrust Joint Manipulation to the XXX spine, I would routinely perform additional medical history screening."

The key point from the survey was that therapists in the US do not believe TJM for the cervical spine to be as safe and efficacious as that for the lumbar and thoracic spines. Further, they are more likely to perform additional screening, abstain from and/or not feel comfortable performing TJM for the cervical spine. These findings revealed a discrepancy between utilization of TJM in the different spinal regions. It remains consistent with the perceptions held by most educators of TJM interventions.

We hope that the findings of the survey and the discussion on the risks of serious complications associated with TJM in this chapter can provide an opportunity for therapists to reconsider the value of TJM interventions in addressing pain and disability in all regions of the spine.

I regularly provide Thrust Joint Manipulation to the XXX spine where it is clinically indicated

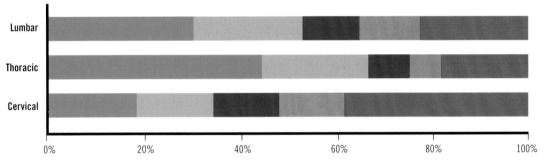

Figure 3.7c: Levels of agreement with the statement "I regularly provide Thrust Joint Manipulation to the XXX spine where it is indicated."

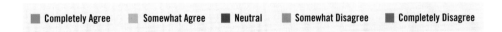

I am comfortable performing Thrust Joint Manipulation to the XXX spine in patients that require it

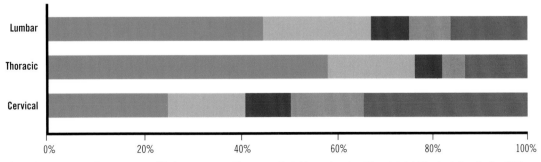

Figure 3.7d: Levels of agreement with the statement "I am comfortable performing Thrust Joint Manipulation to the XXX spine in patients that require it."

3.8: Key Points from Chapter 3

- Thrust joint manipulation to the cervical spine does come with some risks. However, therapists can prevent the occurrences of serious adverse events by conducting a thorough subjective history and objective physical examination and using sound clinical reasoning with the patient before them.

- Serious adverse events can occur in the thoracic spine. Therapists should work to improve their skills in the delivery of TJM to this area of the spine to prevent unwanted side effects as much as serious adverse events.

- The risks associated with TJM in the lumbar spine are negligible. Therapists should consider the risks of worsening of symptoms and disability if their patient can benefit from TJM but it is not provided.

- Therapists in the US believe that TJM is safest and easiest to perform in the thoracic spine.

- It is important for therapists to gain a more evidence-based perspective on risks and benefits associated with TJM to all areas of the spine.

Chapter 3 References

1. Berger S. How safe are the vigorous neck manipulations done by chiropractors? 2014; https://www.washingtonpost.com/national/health-science/how-safe-are-the-vigorous-neck-manipulations-done-by-chiropractors/2014/01/06/26870726-5cf7-11e3-bc56-c6ca94801fac_story.html?utm_term=.9e5672eaec9f. Accessed December 12, 2016.
2. Hayes R. Model Katie May died after chiropractic visit, father says. 2016; http://abc7.com/news/model-katie-may-died-after-chiropractic-visit-father-says/1564102/. Accessed December 4, 2016.
3. Di Fabio RP. Manipulation of the cervical spine: risks and benefits. *Phys Ther.* 1999;79(1):50-65.
4. Haldeman S, Kohlbeck FJ, McGregor M. Stroke, cerebral artery dissection, and cervical spine manipulation therapy. *J Neurol.* 2002;249(8): 1098-1104.
5. Haldeman S, Kohlbeck FJ, McGregor M. Unpredictability of cerebrovascular ischemia associated with cervical spine manipulation therapy: a review of sixty-four cases after cervical spine manipulation. *Spine.* 2002;27(1):49-55.
6. Mann T, Refshauge KM. Causes of complications from cervical spine manipulation. *Aust J Physiother.* 2001;47(4):255-266.
7. Refshauge KM, Parry S, Shirley D, Larsen D, Rivett DA, Boland R. Professional responsibility in relation to cervical spine manipulation. *Aust J Physiother.* 2002;48(3):171-179; discussion 180-175.
8. Terrett AG. Misuse of the literature by medical authors in discussing spinal manipulative therapy injury. *J Manipulative Physiol Ther.* 1995;18(4):203-210.
9. Ernst E. Manipulation of the cervical spine: a systematic review of case reports of serious adverse events, 1995-2001. *Med J Aust.* 2002;176(8): 376-380.
10. Ernst E. Adverse effects of spinal manipulation: a systematic review. *J R Soc Med.* 2007;100(7): 330-338.
11. Puentedura EJ, March J, Anders J, et al. Safety of cervical spine manipulation: are adverse events preventable and are manipulations being performed appropriately? A review of 134 case reports. *J Man Manip Ther.* 2011.
12. Carnes D, Mullinger B, Underwood M. Defining adverse events in manual therapies: a modified Delphi consensus study. *Man Ther.* 2010;15(1):2-6.
13. Senstad O, Leboeuf-Yde C, Borchgrevink C. Frequency and characteristics of side effects of spinal manipulative therapy. *Spine.* 1997;22(4): 435-440; discussion 440-431.
14. Adams G, Sim J. A survey of UK manual therapists' practice of and attitudes towards manipulation and its complications. *Physiother Res Int.* 1998;3(3): 206-227.
15. Assendelft WJ, Bouter LM, Knipschild PG. Complications of spinal manipulation: a comprehensive review of the literature. *J Fam Pract.* 1996;42(5):475-480.
16. Bayerl JR, Buchmuller HR, Pohlmann-Eden B. [Side effects and contraindications of manual therapy in the area of the cervical spine]. *Nervenarzt.* 1985;56(4):194-199.
17. Cagnie B, Vinck E, Beernaert A, Cambier D. How common are side effects of spinal manipulation and can these side effects be predicted? *Man Ther.* 2004;9(3):151-156.
18. Dagenais S, Moher D. Re: Hurwitz EL, Morgenstern H, Vassilaki M, Chiang LM. Frequency and clinical predictors of adverse reactions to chiropractic care in the UCLA neck pain study. Spine 2005; 30: 1477-84. *Spine.* 2006;31(2):253; author reply 253-254.
19. Giles LG. Re: Hurwitz EL, Morgenstern H, Vassilaki M, Chiang L-M. Frequency and clinical predictors of adverse reactions to chiropractic care in the UCLA neck pain study. Spine 2005;30: 1477-84. *Spine.* 2006;31(2):250-251; author reply 251.
20. Grier AR. Adverse reactions to chiropractic treatment and their effects on satisfaction and clinical outcomes among patients enrolled in the UCLA Neck Pain Study. *J Manipulative Physiol Ther.* 2004;27(6):430; author reply 430.
21. Haneline MT, Cooperstein R. Re: Hurwitz et al. Frequency and clinical predictors of adverse reactions to chiropractic care in the UCLA neck pain study. Spine 2005; 30: 1477-84. *Spine.* 2006;31(2):254; author reply 254-255.
22. Hurwitz EL, Morgenstern H, Vassilaki M, Chiang LM. Adverse reactions to chiropractic treatment and their effects on satisfaction and clinical outcomes among patients enrolled in the UCLA Neck Pain Study. *J Manipulative Physiol Ther.* 2004;27(1):16-25.
23. Hurwitz EL, Morgenstern H, Vassilaki M, Chiang LM. Frequency and clinical predictors of adverse reactions to chiropractic care in the UCLA neck pain study. *Spine.* 2005;30(13):1477-1484.
24. Krippendorf DJ. Re: Hurwitz EL, Morgenstern H, Vassilaki M, Chiang LM. Frequency and clinical predictors of adverse reactions to chiropractic care in the UCLA neck pain study. Spine 2005; 30: 1477-84. *Spine.* 2006;31(2):251-252; author reply 252-253.
25. Leboeuf-Yde C, Hennius B, Rudberg E, Leufvenmark P, Thunman M. Side effects of chiropractic treatment: a prospective study. *J Manipulative Physiol Ther.* 1997;20(8):511-515.
26. Powell FC, Hanigan WC, Olivero WC. A risk/benefit analysis of spinal manipulation therapy for relief of lumbar or cervical pain. *Neurosurgery.* 1993;33(1):73-78; discussion 78-79.

27. Rosner AL. Adverse reactions to chiropractic care in the UCLA neck pain study: a response. *J Manipulative Physiol Ther*. 2006;29(3):248-251.

28. Hurwitz EL, Aker PD, Adams AH, Meeker WC, Shekelle PG. Manipulation and mobilization of the cervical spine. A systematic review of the literature. *Spine*. 1996;21(15):1746-1759; discussion 1759-1760.

29. Grant R. Vertebral artery testing - the Australian Physiotherapy Association Protocol after 6 years. *Man Ther*. 1996;1(3):149-153.

30. Rivett DA. The pre-manipulative vertebral artery testing protocol: a brief review. *New Zealand Journal of Physiotherapy* 1995;1:9 - 12.

31. Barker S, Kesson M, Ashmore J, Turner G, Conway J, Stevens D. Professional issue. Guidance for pre-manipulative testing of the cervical spine. *Man Ther*. 2000;5(1):37-40.

32. Licht PB, Christensen HW, Hoilund-Carlsen PF. Is there a role for premanipulative testing before cervical manipulation? *J Manipulative Physiol Ther*. 2000;23(3):175-179.

33. Bolton PS, Stick PE, Lord RS. Failure of clinical tests to predict cerebral ischemia before neck manipulation. *J Manipulative Physiol Ther*. 1989;12(4):304-307.

34. Cote P, Kreitz BG, Cassidy JD, Thiel H. The validity of the extension-rotation test as a clinical screening procedure before neck manipulation: a secondary analysis. *J Manipulative Physiol Ther*. 1996;19(3):159-164.

35. Haldeman S, Kohlbeck FJ, McGregor M. Risk factors and precipitating neck movements causing vertebrobasilar artery dissection after cervical trauma and spinal manipulation. *Spine*. 1999;24(8):785-794.

36. Jull G. Use of high and low velocity cervical manipulative therapy procedures by Australian manipulative physiotherapists. *Aust J Physiother*. 2002;48(3):189-193.

37. Cassidy JD, Lopes AA, Yong-Hing K. The immediate effect of manipulation versus mobilization on pain and range of motion in the cervical spine: a randomized controlled trial. *J Manipulative Physiol Ther*. 1992;15(9):570-575.

38. Nilsson N, Christensen HW, Hartvigsen J. The effect of spinal manipulation in the treatment of cervicogenic headache. *J Manipulative Physiol Ther*. 1997;20(5):326-330.

39. Rothwell DM, Bondy SJ, Williams JI. Chiropractic manipulation and stroke: a population-based case-control study. *Stroke*. 2001;32(5):1054-1060.

40. Bodensteiner JB. Editorial comment: Stroke following chiropractic manipulation. *Semin Pediatr Neurol*. 2014;21(2):127-128.

41. Cassidy JD, Boyle E, Cote P, Hogg-Johnson S, Bondy SJ, Haldeman S. Risk of Carotid Stroke after Chiropractic Care: A Population-Based Case-Crossover Study. *J Stroke Cerebrovasc Dis*. 2016.

42. Cassidy JD, Boyle E, Cote P, et al. Risk of vertebrobasilar stroke and chiropractic care: results of a population-based case-control and case-crossover study. *J Manipulative Physiol Ther*. 2009;32(2 Suppl):S201-208.

43. Thomas LC, Rivett DA, Attia JR, Parsons M, Levi C. Risk factors and clinical features of craniocervical arterial dissection. *Man Ther*. 2011;16(4):351-356.

44. Thomas LC, Rivett DA, Attia JR, Levi C. Risk Factors and Clinical Presentation of Cervical Arterial Dissection: Preliminary Results of a Prospective Case-Control Study. *J Orthop Sports Phys Ther*. 2015;45(7):503-511.

45. Taylor AJ, Kerry R. Neck pain and headache as a result of internal carotid artery dissection: implications for manual therapists. *Manual Therapy*. 2005;10(1):73-77.

46. Taylor AJ, Kerry R. Vascular profiling: Should manual therapists take blood pressure? *Manual Therapy*. 2013;18(4):351-353.

47. Taylor AJ, Kerry R. The 'vertebral artery test'. *Manual Therapy*. 2005;10(4):297.

48. Kerry R, Taylor AJ. Cervical arterial dysfunction assessment and manual therapy. *Manual Therapy*. 2006;11(4):243-253.

49. Taylor AJ, Kerry R. Challenging editorial wisdom and raising the "VBI" debate. *Manual Therapy*. 2008;13(3):e5.

50. Kerry R, Taylor AJ, Mitchell J, McCarthy C. Cervical arterial dysfunction and manual therapy: A critical literature review to inform professional practice. *Manual Therapy*. 2008;13(4):278-288.

51. Puentedura EJ, Slaughter R, Reilly S, Ventura E, Young D. Thrust joint manipulation utilization by U.S. physical therapists. *Journal of Manual & Manipulative Therapy*. 2016:1-15.

52. Cleland JA, Glynn P, Whitman JM, Eberhart SL, MacDonald C, Childs JD. Short-term effects of thrust versus nonthrust mobilization/manipulation directed at the thoracic spine in patients with neck pain: a randomized clinical trial. *Phys Ther*. 2007;87(4):431-440.

53. Cleland JA, Childs JD, Fritz JM, Whitman JM, Eberhart SL. Development of a clinical prediction rule for guiding treatment of a subgroup of patients with neck pain: use of thoracic spine manipulation, exercise, and patient education. *Phys Ther*. 2007;87(1):9-23.

54. Cleland JA, Childs JD, McRae M, Palmer JA, Stowell T. Immediate effects of thoracic manipulation in patients with neck pain: a randomized clinical trial. *Man Ther*. 2005;10(2):127-135.

55. Cleland JA, Mintken PE, Carpenter K, et al. Examination of a clinical prediction rule to identify patients with neck pain likely to benefit from thoracic spine thrust manipulation and a general cervical range of motion exercise: multi-center randomized clinical trial. *Phys Ther*. 2010;90(9):1239-1250.

56. Mintken PE, Cleland JA, Carpenter KJ, Bieniek ML, Keirns M, Whitman JM. Some factors predict successful short-term outcomes in individuals with shoulder pain receiving cervicothoracic manipulation: a single-arm trial. *Phys Ther*. 2010;90(1):26-42.

57. Rhon DI, Boyles RE, Cleland JA, Brown DL. A manual physical therapy approach versus subacromial corticosteroid injection for treatment of shoulder impingement syndrome: a protocol for a randomised clinical trial. *BMJ Open*. 2011;1(2):e000137.

58. Gonzalez-Iglesias J, Cleland JA, Neto F, Hall T, Fernandez-de-las-Penas C. Mobilization with movement, thoracic spine manipulation, and dry needling for the management of temporomandibular disorder: a prospective case series. *Physiother Theory Pract*. 2013;29(8):586-595.

59. Puentedura EJ, O'Grady WH. Safety of thrust joint manipulation in the thoracic spine: a systematic review. *J Man Manip Ther*. 2015;23(3):154-161.

60. Frost H, Lamb SE, Doll HA, Carver PT, Stewart-Brown S. Randomised controlled trial of physiotherapy compared with advice for low back pain. *BMJ*. 2004;329(7468):708.

61. Haldeman S, Rubinstein SM. Cauda equina syndrome in patients undergoing manipulation of the lumbar spine. *Spine*. 1992;17(12):1469-1473.

62. Hebert JJ, Stomski NJ, French SD, Rubinstein SM. Serious Adverse Events and Spinal Manipulative Therapy of the Low Back Region: A Systematic Review of Cases. *J Manipulative Physiol Ther*. 2015;38(9):677-691.

63. Shekelle PG, Adams AH, Chassin MR, Hurwitz EL, Brook RH. Spinal manipulation for low-back pain. Annals of internal medicine. 1992;117(7):590-598.

64. Bronfort G. Spinal manipulation: current state of research and its indications. *Neurol Clin*. 1999;17(1):91-111.

65. Tannenbaum H, Davis P, Russell AS, et al. An evidence-based approach to prescribing NSAIDs in musculoskeletal disease: a Canadian consensus. Canadian NSAID Consensus Participants. *CMAJ*. 1996;155(1):77-88.

66. Tamblyn R, Berkson L, Dauphinee WD, et al. Unnecessary prescribing of NSAIDs and the management of NSAID-related gastropathy in medical practice. *Ann Intern Med*. 1997;127(6): 429-438.

67. Hungin AP, Kean WF. Nonsteroidal anti-inflammatory drugs: overused or underused in osteoarthritis? *Am J Med*. 2001;110(1A):8S-11S.

68. Albert CM, Mittleman MA, Chae CU, Lee IM, Hennekens CH, Manson JE. Triggering of sudden death from cardiac causes by vigorous exertion. *N Engl J Med*. 2000;343(19):1355-1361.

69. Nadler SF, Prybicien M, Malanga GA, Sicher D. Complications from therapeutic modalities: results of a national survey of athletic trainers. *Arch Phys Med Rehabil*. 2003;84(6):849-853.

70. Childs JD, Flynn TW, Fritz JM. A perspective for considering the risks and benefits of spinal manipulation in patients with low back pain. *Manual therapy*. 2006;11(4):316-320.

71. Fritz JM, George SZ. Identifying psychosocial variables in patients with acute work-related low back pain: the importance of fear-avoidance beliefs. *Phys Ther*. 2002;82(10):973-983.

72. Frank JW, Brooker A, DeMaio SE, et al. Disability resulting from occupational low back pain. Part 11: What do we know about secondary prevention ? A review of the scientific evidence on prevention after disability begins. *Spine*. 1996;21:2918-2929.

73. Hashemi L, Webster BS, Clancy EA, Volinn E. Length of disability and cost of workers' compensation low back pain claims. *J Occup Environ Med*. 1997;39(10):937-945.

74. Hiebert R, Skovron ML, Nordin M, Crane M. Work restrictions and outcome of nonspecific low back pain. *Spine (Phila Pa 1976)*. 2003;28(7):722-728.

75. Waddell G. Chiropractic for low back pain. Evidence for manipulation is stronger than that for most orthodox medical treatments. *BMJ*. 1999;318(7178):262.

76. Noteboom JT, Little C, Boissonnault W. Thrust joint manipulation curricula in first-professional physical therapy education: 2012 update. *J Orthop Sports Phys Ther*. 2015;45(6):471-476.

77. Boissonnault W, Bryan JM, Fox KJ. Joint manipulation curricula in physical therapist professional degree programs. *J Orthop Sports Phys Ther*. 2004;34(4):171-178; discussion 179-181.

Chapter 4

Clinical Reasoning and Thrust Joint Manipulation

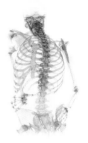

4.1: Chapter Objectives

How does one, or more correctly, how *should* one decide when to use thrust joint manipulation (TJM) in the management of their patient? As we have seen in the last chapter, clinicians should carefully and thoroughly look for any reason *not* to use TJM with their patient. Prevention of serious adverse events and unwanted side effects associated with the provision of TJM in the spine is vital. Screening for contraindications and precautions, and performing a thorough examination is the starting point. However, the clinician should also use sound clinical reasoning when determining if they will use TJM techniques.

After considering the research evidence for the effectiveness and safety of TJM in the spine, it may appear as though there are many more reasons not to manipulate a patient's spine than there might be to do so. How we decide to use TJM should involve the use of sound clinical reasoning. In this chapter, we will explore the clinical reasoning process and how we might apply it to the provision of TJM in our patients with spinal dysfunction.

4.2: Defining Clinical Reasoning

Clinical reasoning is the thinking that underlies a clinician's decision process. It has been defined as the process by which a clinician, interacting with their patient, will structure meaning, goals and health management strategies based on clinical data, the patient's wishes, values and choices, and professional judgement and knowledge.[1] Without it, clinical practice would just be a technical operation that requires direction from a 'decision maker.' In that sense, clinical reasoning is the foundation of professional clinical practice. Understanding clinical reasoning will improve the clinician's own thinking through patient problems and broaden the repertoire of clinical patterns that he or she recognizes.

The main aim of the clinical reasoning process is to arrive at the answers to the following five basic questions that all clinicians should be asking:

1. What is the source of the patient's symptoms and/or dysfunction?

2. Are there any contributing factors?

3. What are the contraindications and precautions to physical examination and treatment (if any)?

4. What is the prognosis?

5. What treatment interventions should be selected and what progression is most likely?

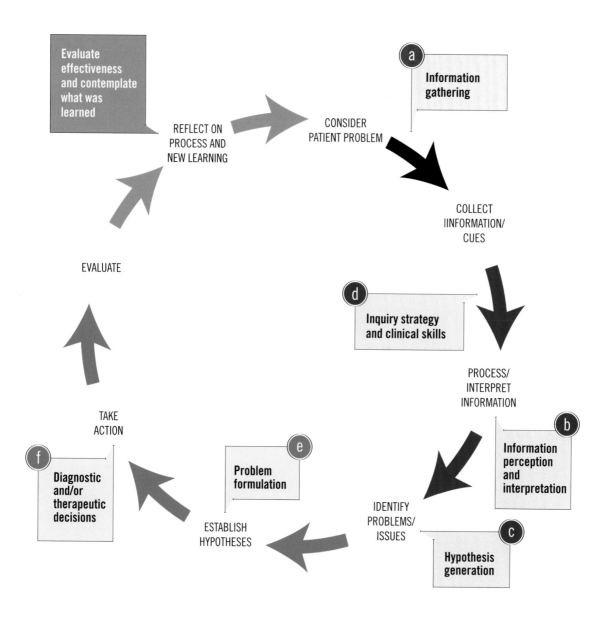

Figure 4.2a: The clinical reasoning cycle. Adapted from Levett-Jones et al.[2]

By searching for the answers to these questions, the clinician must apply relevant knowledge (facts, procedures, concepts and principles) and clinical skills in the evaluation, diagnosis and management of their patient's problem. The clinical reasoning process describes the steps taken by clinicians to reach diagnostic and management decisions.

Researchers who have focused on clinical reasoning have described it as a cyclical and interactive process involving: a) information gathering; b) information perception and interpretation; c) hypothesis generation; d) inquiry strategy and clinical skills; e) problem formulation; and f) diagnostic and/or therapeutic decisions (Figure 4.2a).

An important step often omitted is the evaluation or assessment of outcomes from the process. This is where the clinician should take the time to evaluate the effectiveness of their reasoning process, and to contemplate what was learned and what should be done differently (if necessary) next time. Of course, this requires time and is one of the many factors that can influence a clinician's clinical reasoning skills. Other factors that will influence those skills include a mixture of external and internal factors, which relate to the specifics of the task, the setting, the patient and the clinician. The critical factors pertaining to the clinician include their cognitive skills, metacognitive skills and knowledge base.

Cognitive skills refer to the thinking processes of the clinician such as data analysis and synthesis, and the inquiry strategies such as hypothesis testing. In other words, it is making sense of what the patient is saying

about their problem and having a strategy to test what might be a reasonable source of the problem. The cognitive skills and knowledge base of the clinician are interdependent because the inquiry strategy of hypothesis testing is said to play a significant role in the acquisition of knowledge.[3,4] Errors in clinical reasoning are frequently related to errors in cognition, for example, overemphasis on findings that support an existing hypothesis, or misinterpreting non-contributory information as confirming an existing hypothesis.[3] A very common error is to focus too much on a favored hypothesis, and many clinicians are aware of the danger of preoccupation with one diagnosis, one structure or one system at the expense of the others.

Metacognition refers to a clinician's awareness and ability to think about their thinking. Experienced clinicians are able to recognize and respond appropriately to relevant cues, even without explicit awareness of their own reasoning. This has been referred to as 'knowing-in-action.'[5] Expertise is said to be reached through clinical experience where reasoning involves 'reflection-in-action' and 'reflection-about-action.' 'Reflection-in-action' refers to thinking about what you are doing while you do it, i.e. conducting a 'reflective conversation' with yourself.[5] 'Reflection-about-action' refers to thinking about what you were doing after you have done it, i.e. reviewing what happened in practice.[5] By promoting awareness, reflection and critical appraisal, a clinician will be able to recognize clinical patterns in the more complex presentations and acquire new clinical patterns not previously appreciated. In this way, clinical outcomes can be better understood and improved upon.

Knowledge is what all clinicians initially gain through their respective training programs, but also build upon through experience and clinical practice. Expertise and diagnostic accuracy in clinical reasoning are dependent upon a clinician's knowledge in a particular area.[6] It is not simply how much a clinician knows, but more about the organization of that knowledge. Clinicians need to keep in perspective what they need to know in clinical practice versus what might be nice, marginal or irrelevant to know. There is also a difference between biomedical knowledge and clinical knowledge. Biomedical knowledge is what is known or believed in the basic sciences such as anatomy, biomechanics, pathoanatomy, pathobiomechanics, pathophysiology, psychology, and pain mechanisms and healing. Clinical knowledge refers to the clinical patterns and the 'if/then' guides to actions which clinicians use on a day-to-day basis with or without a sound biomechanical basis. It is what a clinician has found to 'work' for them in clinical practice. Optimal patient care should emerge as the clinician integrates both clinical and biomedical knowledge.[6]

We should all strive to be 'thinking clinicians' who question, explore and reflect in order to improve our clinical reasoning skills. To achieve this, we need to increase awareness of our reasoning processes, and broaden our perspective beyond diagnostic reasoning. We should develop a greater awareness of our reasoning errors and encourage the use of alternative inquiry strategies and hypothesis testing to prove/disprove our favored hypotheses. This requires us to find the time for regular reflection about our clinical reasoning and practice patterns.

4.3: Clinical Reasoning Models for Thrust Joint Manipulation

While scientific validation for the use of TJM remains somewhat limited across the broad spectrum of patients that clinicians will likely encounter, it is very encouraging to see research evidence begin to support its use in certain subgroups of patients. Remembering that evidence-based practice involves more than just the best of available research evidence, we can draw upon evidence from clinical experience and the values and preferences of our patients. Using the best of available research evidence might have us considering the application of a clinical prediction rule, or perhaps a well-supported clinical practice guideline. Using the best of available clinical expertise might have us use TJM in particular clinical presentations we have seen before on numerous occasions, where outcomes have been favorable. Finally, using the best of the values and preferences from our patients might have us avoiding the use of TJM where there has been an unfavorable experience with it in their past. Alternatively, we may decide to use TJM where the patient reports favorable experiences with it in the past.

We contend that there are five ways to consider TJM in a clinical reasoning approach. A research evidence approach, a biomechanical approach, a neurophysiological approach, a patient expectation (placebo) approach, and a pain neuroscience education (PNE) approach. The latter four approaches may be considered as falling under the mantle of theoretical constructs and biological plausibility.

4.4: Research Evidence in Clinical Reasoning

A review of chapter two of this book should remind us that while the bulk of the current evidence available for the effectiveness of TJM to the spine is only moderate at best, this may have more to do with the way that research was conducted than the true effectiveness of TJM. There is good evidence for sub-grouping patients with low back and neck pain who are more likely to respond favorably to the addition of TJM in their treatment package. A clinical prediction rule for patients with low back pain who are more likely to benefit from TJM has been validated and may assist clinicians in their reasoning process. While not yet validated, there is also a clinical prediction rule for patients with neck pain who will respond favorably to TJM to their cervical spine. Also, there is strong evidence that patients with neck pain may benefit from TJM to their thoracic spine, as long as there are no contraindications.

It is important to remember that clinical prediction rules do not replace sound clinical reasoning, and sound clinical reasoning requires a thorough subjective history and physical examination. If, after completing a detailed history and physical examination, it becomes apparent that a patient meets the clinical prediction rule for TJM to their lumbar spine, do not forget to consider the patient's values and preferences as well as the clinical experience/expertise of the clinician. It is quite possible that such a patient, who meets the rule, may not be considered a good candidate for TJM because of an unfavorable past experience with TJM or other patient-related factors beyond those accounted for in the rule. Equally, a patient may not meet the rule but report favorable past experiences with TJM and other patient-related factors that suggest TJM may be reasonably considered.

In general, it appears that patients presenting with more acute symptoms (shorter duration), localized rather than widespread areas of symptoms, joint hypomobility rather than hypermobility, low fear avoidance beliefs, and *without* negative expectations or beliefs about TJM will tend to benefit from its inclusion in a treatment program.

4.5: Biomechanical Effects in Clinical Reasoning

From a historical aspect, TJM has been seen as a treatment technique designed to restore or improve range of motion (ROM) within the manipulated joint(s). Nansel et al[7] used goniometry to compare cervical ROM pre- and post-manipulation in a sample of 24 asymptomatic subjects who exhibited asymmetrical loss of lateral flexion range (10° or greater). They reported a significant increase in cervical ROM for a four-hour time period after TJM to the lower cervical spine when compared to subjects who received placebo manipulation.[7] In another study involving 16 patients with chronic neck pain, cervical ROM and pain pressure thresholds (PPT) were measured before and after thrust manipulation to the C5/6 and C6/7 levels.[8] Results from that study found that both cervical ROM and PPT increased significantly following the manipulation.[8]

Cassidy et al[9] examined for cervical ROM changes following a single rotational manipulation in 52 subjects suffering from unilateral neck pain with referral into the trapezius muscle. The authors found an immediate increase in cervical ROM recorded in three planes following the manipulation; however, they found a similar increase (no significant difference) in ROM with non-thrust mobilization treatment applied to a second group of 48 subjects. While the results of this study support the notion that TJM leads to restoration or improvement in ROM, it demonstrated that similar changes in ROM might be achieved through non-thrust mobilization.

In contrast, Martinez-Segura et al[10] reported on the immediate effects on active cervical ROM after a single spine TJM versus a mobilization procedure. In their study, 70 patients with mechanical neck pain (25 males; age 20 – 55) were randomized to receive a TJM or non-thrust mobilization technique. Active ROM was assessed pre-treatment and five minutes post-treatment by an assessor blinded to the treatment allocation. Results indicated that the TJM group obtained greater improvement in ROM than the mobilization group (p<0.001).[10] From these studies on the effects of TJM to the cervical spine, it could be argued that there is some evidence for its effectiveness on active ROM, at least in the short term.

Some definitions of spinal TJM suggest that the procedure itself takes the joints beyond the normal ROM and into the "paraphysiological" ROM[11,12] and thereby causes the audible release or cavitation. If this was so, then it would follow that ROM immediately following a TJM should show a significant increase. However, Klein et al[13] reported on a descriptive study involving 14 asymptomatic volunteers whereby ROM was measured by a 3D electrogoniometer during the TJM. The authors recorded the pattern of motion and the amplitudes obtained during TJM on two levels (C3 and C5) and on the left and right sides.

The subjects received seated cervical rotation/lateral flexion TJM. The mean ROM recorded were 30° (SD = 9°) for axial rotation, 46° (SD = 8°) for lateral bending and 2° (SD = 10°) for flexion.[13] The findings indicated that, for the specific TJM technique investigated, maximal amplitude between the head and trunk did not exceed physiological ROM. The study examined total ROM excursion between the head and trunk but did not assess for motion at specific intervertebral segments or zygapophyseal (facet) joints. It has been suggested that TJM produces unique facet joint capsule strain patterns[14], which might explain the biomechanical response of the technique.

Cascioli et al[15] reported on a study using computed tomography (CT) and plain film radiography to analyze the size and density of cervical facet joint spaces in asymptomatic subjects before and after TJM. Twenty-two subjects underwent pre- and post-TJM imaging. The authors found no significant change in the width, area, and density values of the facet joint spaces immediately after the cervical TJM.[15] They concluded that there was no evidence of gas in the joint space or obvious increase in facet joint space width immediately after CSM, which was not consistent with the prevailing understanding of cavitation in joints.[15]

Cramer et al[16] investigated the effects of TJM on gapping of zygapophyseal joints. Sixteen healthy student volunteers had anterior to posterior measurements of their zygapophyseal joints from MRI scans taken before and after side-lying TJM to the lumbar spine. They found that subjects who were left in side-lying for imaging after the TJM technique demonstrated the greatest increase in gapping (0.7 mm vs. 0.0 mm for controls).[16]

A review of the literature would therefore suggest that there are some biomechanical effects associated with TJM, but the exact mechanisms remain largely unexplained. Evidence suggests that TJM causes vertebral movement, gapping of facet joints, and increased intervertebral motion. However, the changes observed do not last long, are not site or joint-level specific, and there are no observed changes in spinal alignment or vertebral position.

From the clinical reasoning point of view, clinicians could consider it appropriate to use TJM to achieve a temporary increase in intervertebral motion; to gap a presumed symptomatic facet joint; or to cause passive vertebral movement, which may allow a patient to move on to active exercises and movement. TJM is therefore used as a small but perhaps important part of a more comprehensive rehabilitation approach.

4.6: Neurophysiologic Effects in Clinical Reasoning

The neurophysiologic mechanisms by which TJM techniques are effective have yet to be fully understood, and both segmental and central mechanisms have been proposed.[17] It is thought that the reduction in pain and reduced muscle tone observed following spinal TJM may involve reflex inhibition of pain or reflex muscle relaxation mediated through joint mechanoreceptors.[18] TJM is thought to specifically target the facet joints which are highly innervated and contain numerous mechanoreceptors.[19-22] It has been proposed that TJM techniques to the spine may beneficially stimulate these mechanoreceptors and thereby alter aberrant sensory input.[18]

Coronado et al[23] completed a systematic review and meta-analysis of changes in pain sensitivity following TJM. From 997 articles identified, 20 met their inclusion criteria for review and meta-analysis. TJM demonstrated a favorable effect over other interventions on increasing pain pressure thresholds (PPT). Subgroup analysis showed a significant effect of TJM on increasing PPT at the remote sites of stimulus application supporting a potential central nervous system mechanism.

A few studies have used double-blind controls and placebo groups to compare the therapeutic effects of TJM to either a sham manipulation or a minimal contact intervention. In these studies, the sympathetic nervous system response to TJM is measured by skin conductance, with increased conductance signifying an excitatory response. Hypoalgesia is measured as an increase in mechanical pain pressure threshold (PPT). In a review of a potential neurophysiological mechanism for post-manipulation hypoalgesia, Wright[24] argued that the analgesic response to spinal TJM is likely the result of the stimulation of mechanoreceptors that provide afferent input to the central nervous system which then triggers descending pain inhibitory pathways originating from the periaqueductal grey area of the midbrain (PAG).

In a study involving 30 healthy subjects, Fernandez-de-las-Penas et al[17] examined the effects of C7/T1 TJM on PPT over bilateral C5/6 facet joints. The subjects were randomized to receive a TJM to C7/T1 on their upper extremity dominant side, a TJM to C7/T1 on their non-dominant side, or a sham-manual procedure. The outcome measure was PPT on over right and left C5/6 facet joints, which was assessed pre-intervention and five minutes post-intervention by an assessor blinded to the intervention allocation of the subjects. Their results demonstrated that TJM to either side resulted in greater improvements in PPT over both right and left C5/6 facet joints than the sham-manual procedure (p<0.05).[17]

Ruiz-Saez et al[25] reported on changes in PPT over latent myofascial trigger points in the upper trapezius muscle after a C3 through C4 'upslope' TJM in pain-free subjects. The study involved 72 healthy volunteers (46 women; mean age 31 years, SD 10 years) who were screened for the presence of myofascial trigger points in their upper trapezius and intervertebral joint dysfunction at the C3 through C4 level assessed by the lateral gliding test for the cervical spine. Subjects were randomly assigned to receive the TJM or a sham manual procedure. Analysis of variance showed an interaction between group and time (F = 37.240; p<0.001), with the experimental group showing a trend toward an increase in PPT levels after the TJM procedure, and the control group showing a trend toward a decrease in PPT.[25] The authors concluded that a TJM directed at the C3 through C4 segment induced changes in PPT in latent myofascial trigger points in the upper trapezius muscle.

Fernandez-Carnero et al[26] reported on a repeated-measures, crossover, single-blinded randomized study involving 10 patients with lateral epicondylalgia. The patients were administered either a single TJM to the cervical spine or a manual contact intervention (sham manipulation). PPT, hot and cold pain pressure thresholds (HPT and CPT, respectively) and pain-free grip force (PGF) were compared pre-intervention and five minutes post-intervention. Their analysis demonstrated that the application of TJM to the cervical spine produced an immediate bilateral increase in PPT, and increased PGF on the affected side in patients with lateral epicondylalgia.[26]

Haavik-Taylor and Murphy[27] reported on a study investigating the immediate sensorimotor neurophysiological effects of TJM using somatosensory evoked potentials (SEPs). Twenty-four subjects with a history of recurring neck stiffness and/or neck pain, but with no acute symptoms at the time of the study were randomly assigned to receive a single session of cervical TJM, or passive head movement. Spinal (N11, N13) brainstem (P14) and cortical (N20, N30) SEPs to median nerve stimulation were recorded before and for 30 minutes after either intervention. Significant findings were for decreased amplitude of parietal N20 and frontal N20 SEP components following the TJM compared to pre-manipulation baseline values.[27] The authors concluded that TJM of dysfunctional cervical joints can lead to transient cortical plastic changes (altered cortical somatosensory processing and sensorimotor integration), as demonstrated by the attenuation of cortical SEPs.[27]

Teodorczyk-Injeyan et al[28] investigated the effect of a single thoracic spine TJM on the in vitro production of inflammatory cytokines - tumor necrosis factor alpha (TNF-α), and interleukin 1Beta(IL-1Beta) - in relation to the systemic (in vivo) levels of neurotransmitter substance P (SP). They assigned 64 asymptomatic subjects to receive thoracic TJM, sham manipulation, or no manual contact (control). Blood and serum samples were obtained from all subjects before and then at 20 minutes and two hours after intervention. Over the study period, a significant proportion ($p \leq 0.05$) of the sham and control subjects had progressive increases in the synthesis of pro-inflammatory cytokines TNF-α and IL-1Beta, whereas the production of both cytokines decreased gradually in subjects receiving thoracic TJM.[28] In all groups, serum levels of SP remained unchanged within two hours after intervention. They concluded that the subjects receiving thoracic TJM had a time-dependent attenuation of lipopolysaccharide-induced production of inflammatory cytokines which was unrelated to systemic levels of substance P.

In a prospective, blinded study, Degenhardt et al[29] examined the effects of spinal TJM on levels of circulatory pain biomarkers in 20 subjects (10 with chronic LBP and 10 controls without LBP). Blood was collected for five consecutive days and on the fourth day, spinal TJM was administered to all subjects one hour before blood collection. They found increases from baseline in beta-endorphin and N-palmitoylethanolamide (PEA) levels and a decrease in anandemide (arachidonoylethanolamide [AEA]) levels immediately post treatment for both groups. Subgroup analysis showed that subjects with chronic LBP had significantly reduced 5-hyrdoxyindoleacetic acid (5-HIAA) levels at 30 minutes post treatment ($p=0.05$) and serotonin (5-hydroxytryptamine [5-HT]) levels at 24 hours post treatment ($p=0.02$) when compared with baseline concentrations.[29]

Although only a small pilot study, the authors were able to demonstrate that spinal TJM led to an increase in beta-endorphins (which would presumably decrease pain) in subjects with chronic LBP as well as in asymptomatic subjects. There was also a reduction in pain biomarkers (5-HIAA and 5-HT) in subjects with chronic LBP as well as in symptomatic subjects. Interestingly, the degree and duration of the changes in circulatory pain biomarkers were greater in subjects with chronic LBP than in controls.[29]

Bishop et al[30] reported on a randomized laboratory study involving 90 healthy volunteers who were assigned to receive one of three interventions (TJM, exercise, or rest) to the upper thoracic spine. They collected experimental pain sensitivity measures of cervical and lumbar innervated areas before and immediately after the interventions. While no interactions or intervention (group) effects were noted for pressure or A-delta-mediated thermal pain responses, participants who received TJM had greater reductions in temporal sensory summation. Their finding of reduced temporal sensory summation has potentially meaningful implications. Patients with chronic pain conditions often demonstrate increased rates and magnitudes of temporal sensory summation when compared with pain-free individuals. They speculated that an intervention like TJM that reduces temporal sensory summation may inhibit or reduce the potential for central sensitization in maintaining musculoskeletal pain.[30]

From the studies cited above, the evidence suggests that spinal TJM causes improvement in local chemistry; decrease in pro-inflammatory cytokines; increase in local endorphins; and reduction in temporal sensory summation, all of which would appear to provide beneficial clinical effects. However, the evidence also suggests that the changes do not appear to be long-lasting and are systemic in nature and not specific to the area or focus of joint manipulation.

From the clinical reasoning point of view, clinicians could consider it appropriate to use TJM to achieve temporary improvements in local chemistry, decrease in pro-inflammatory cytokines, and increase in local endorphins. All of these would likely provide an immediate though temporary relief in nociception and pain, which may allow a patient to move on to active exercises and movement. Once again, TJM may be used as a small but perhaps important part of a more comprehensive rehabilitation approach.

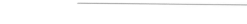

4.7: Patient Expectation in Clinical Reasoning

In a recent narrative review article, Bialosky et al[31] proposed a more comprehensive model of the proposed biomechanical and/or neurophysiological mechanisms of spinal TJM. They noted that a limitation of the current literature was the failure to acknowledge the potential for a combined effect of these mechanisms, and also to account for the non-specific mechanisms associated with spinal TJM in the treatment of musculoskeletal pain. A number of neurophysiological responses associated with spinal TJM are also associated with non-specific effects such as placebo, expectation, fear, and catastrophizing.[31] A comprehensive model was proposed which suggests a mechanical stimulus (the TJM technique) initiates a number of potential neurophysiological effects that produce the clinical outcomes associated with TJM in the treatment of musculoskeletal pain.[31] The non-specific effects certainly warrant further investigation.

An important distinction to be made is that placebo is not equivalent to 'nothing,' and yet many research designs attempt to examine outcomes of a treatment by comparing it to a 'placebo' intervention. In those situations, researchers have often used 'no intervention' as the placebo. The word 'placebo' is derived from the Latin "I shall please"[32] and traditionally, when patients participating in studies are given a placebo treatment, they will have a perceived or actual improvement in their condition. This phenomenon is called the 'placebo effect'. In a sense, placebo is a positive expectation that an intervention will help a condition. The patient believes treatment will help them and, therefore, it does. The opposite effect is 'nocebo' and this is a negative expectation that an intervention will not help but rather harm a condition. The patient believes treatment will not help or may actually harm them and, therefore, it does not help or makes their condition worse.

Expectation of benefit (placebo) has been shown to have a robust effect on pain.[33,34] It has also be shown to induce biological changes in central nervous system activation,[35-37] opioid pathways,[38] and dopamine production.[39] Negative expectation has also been shown to have a potent effect. In a recent study, Bingel et al[40] showed how divergent expectations could alter the analgesic efficacy of a potent opioid in healthy volunteers by using brain imaging. They assessed the effect of a fixed concentration of the μ-opioid agonist remifentanil on constant heat pain under three experimental conditions using a within-subject design: with no expectation of analgesia; with expectancy of a positive analgesic effect; and with negative expectancy of analgesia (i.e. expectation of hyperalgesia or exacerbation of pain). Using functional MRI to record brain activity to corroborate the effects of expectations on the analgesic efficacy of the opioid, they found that positive treatment expectancy substantially enhanced (doubled) the analgesic benefit of remifentanil. In contrast, negative treatment expectancy abolished remifentanil analgesia.[40] In this case, a normally potent opioid analgesic was rendered ineffective by negative expectation.

Bishop et al[41] performed secondary analysis of data from a clinical trial of interventions for neck pain. They reviewed expectations of benefit collected prior to interventions in 140 patients and found that general expectations of benefit had a strong influence on clinical outcomes.

These non-specific effects (placebo, expectation) will need to be considered more carefully in all future research on the effects of treatment interventions. In our study on the development of the clinical prediction rule for TJM in patients with neck pain, we collected data from patients on positive or negative expectations of benefit with TJM. A positive expectation that TJM would help their current episode of neck pain came out as one of the four predictors included in the rule. From the clinical reasoning point of view, clinicians could consider it appropriate to use TJM to meet the existing expectations of their patient or enhance outcomes by creating positive expectations. Clinicians should harness the power of non-specific effects of treatment to enhance patient outcomes and encourage advancement to more active exercises and movement. Here too, TJM may be used as part of that more comprehensive rehabilitation approach.

4.8: Pain Neuroscience Education in Clinical Reasoning

Pain neuroscience education (PNE) refers to teaching people with chronic pain about the neurobiology and neurophysiology of their pain.[42] Several controlled trials and two recent systematic reviews have reported favorable outcomes following PNE in patients with chronic pain in terms of reduced pain scores, pain catastrophization, disability, and improved physical performance.[43-48] The focus of PNE is reconceptualization of pain by teaching patients more about the biological and physiological processes involved with their pain experiences versus focusing solely on tissue pathology. In the patient with chronic spine related pain, this reconceptualization attempts to help them understand that their pain and tissue injury are different constructs.[45,49,50]

Because the aim is to shift the patient's focus from the tissues in the spine as the source of their pain to the brain's interpretation of inputs, many clinicians mistakenly believe that PNE should be a 'hands-off,' education-only approach. An argument is made that by providing manual therapy or TJM to address tissue pathology, the patient's focus will be immediately brought back to their spinal tissues as the source of their problem.

Traditionally, TJM is thought to be dependent upon bottom-up-mediated factors like stimulus intensity, but in recent years, greater attention has been drawn to top-down-mediated factors like expectations.[51,52] If we take the case of a patient with low back pain receiving a TJM intervention to their lumbar spine, the mechanical stimulus can cause movement at the spinal motion segments, which may improve segmental motion, decrease local tissue inflammatory factors, and facilitate local muscular control.[28,53,54] The intent is to decrease nociceptive input into the system and thereby modulate the pain experience.

We could consider this a bottom-up approach. But we should also consider the "top down" effects, i.e. the brain and its integral role in producing a pain experience.

When TJM is provided to a patient with chronic spinal pain, it is done with a complex set of physical and psychological stimuli (tactile, verbal and non-verbal cues) which tell the patient that clinical improvement should be happening soon. These stimuli represent the context around the therapy and the patient, and such a context may be as important as the specific effect of the intervention.[42] The contextual factors that might affect the therapeutic outcome can be represented by the characteristics of the treatment (hand contact, direction of movement, force), the patient's and therapist's characteristics (treatment and pain beliefs, status, gender), the patient-provider relationship (suggestion, reassurance, and compassion), and finally, the healthcare setting (clinic and room layout).[55]

Recent research has shown that people with chronic pain demonstrate impairments in laterality judgements (identifying a body part as being oriented to the left or right), which is considered dependent on an intact body schema in the sensorimotor areas of the cortex.[56-59] Furthermore, body image is disrupted, and tactile acuity is decreased in the area of usual pain in patients with chronic pain.[60] This phenomenon has been referred to as 'smudging' of the sensorimotor homunculus[61] and it is thought that retraining laterality and tactile discrimination can 'sharpen' or 'refocus' the homunculus and lead to decreased pain.[62,63] We would argue that the skillful delivery of TJM to the low back motion segments, as long as they do not evoke a pain response, can assist in re-establishing tactile discrimination (can assist in 'localization' of the spinal motion segment) and thereby 'sharpen' or 'refocus' the homunculus. Consider that the skillful delivery of TJM involves constant communication between the patient and clinician, "How does this feel here?", "Can you feel me pressing on your L5 spinous process", "What if I push it this way?" It could be argued that the application of TJM in such a manner would run sensory and proprioceptive neural circuits within the brain and help to refresh its representational body maps.

From the clinical reasoning point of view, clinicians could consider it appropriate to use TJM, as long as it does not evoke a pain response, to reestablish more accurate or focused body schemas within the brain. Of course, TJM would need to be provided within the context of a PNE approach and would play only a minor role in the overall rehabilitation program. A greater focus would be on education, exercise, sleep hygiene, goals, etc.

4.9: Key Points from Chapter 4

- While it is vital to understand when not to use TJM in a patient with spinal pain, it is also important to know when it might be of benefit.

- Clinical reasoning is the cyclic and interactive process that a clinician engages in to learn everything they need to know about their patient's condition and what treatment intervention/approach might help them most.

- The reasons to use TJM in a patient may encompass support from research evidence, or support from theoretical constructs and biological plausibility.

- Clinicians may decide to use TJM for its apparent mechanical, neurophysiologic or expectation-of-benefit effects.

- There is growing support for TJM in a pain neuroscience education approach to patients with chronic spinal pain.

Chapter 4 References

1. Higgs J, Jones MA. Clinical decision making and multiple problem spaces. In: Higgs J, Jones MA, Loftus S, Christensen N, eds. *Clinical reasoning in the health professions*. 3rd ed. Oxford: Butterworth-Heinemann; 2008:3-14.

2. Levett-Jones T, Hoffman K, Dempsey J, et al. The 'five rights' of clinical reasoning: an educational model to enhance nursing students' ability to identify and manage clinically 'at risk' patients. *Nurse Educ Today*. 2010;30(6):515-520.

3. Jones M. Clinical reasoning: the foundation of clinical practice. Part 1. *Aust J Physiother*. 1997;43(3):167-170.

4. Edwards I, Jones M, Carr J, Braunack-Mayer A, Jensen GM. Clinical reasoning strategies in physical therapy. *Phys Ther*. 2004;84(4):312-330; discussion 331-315.

5. Shon D. *The reflective practitioner: How professionals think in action*. New York: Basic Books; 1983.

6. Higgs J, Jones MA, Loftus S, Christensen N. *Clinical reasoning in the health professions*. 3rd ed. Oxford: Butterworth-Heinemann; 2008.

7. Nansel D, Jansen R, Cremata E, Dhami MS, Holley D. Effects of cervical adjustments on lateral-flexion passive end-range asymmetry and on blood pressure, heart rate and plasma catecholamine levels. *J Manipulative Physiol Ther*. 1991;14(8):450-456.

8. Suter E, McMorland G. Decrease in elbow flexor inhibition after cervical spine manipulation in patients with chronic neck pain. *Clin Biomech (Bristol, Avon)*. 2002;17(7):541-544.

9. Cassidy JD, Lopes AA, Yong-Hing K. The immediate effect of manipulation versus mobilization on pain and range of motion in the cervical spine: a randomized controlled trial. *J Manipulative Physiol Ther*. 1992;15(9):570-575.

10. Martinez-Segura R, Fernandez-de-las-Penas C, Ruiz-Saez M, Lopez-Jimenez C, Rodriguez-Blanco C. Immediate effects on neck pain and active range of motion after a single cervical high-velocity low-amplitude manipulation in subjects presenting with mechanical neck pain: a randomized controlled trial. *J Manipulative Physiol Ther*. 2006;29(7):511-517.

11. Sandoz R. Some physical mechanisms and effects of spinal adjustments. *Ann Swiss Chiropractic Assoc*. 1976;6:91-142.

12. Vernon H, Mrozek J. A revised definition of manipulation. *J Manipulative Physiol Ther*. 2005;28(1):68-72.

13. Klein P, Broers C, Feipel V, et al. Global 3D head-trunk kinematics during cervical spine manipulation at different levels. *Clin Biomech (Bristol, Avon)*. 2003;18(9):827-831.

14. Ianuzzi A, Khalsa PS. High loading rate during spinal manipulation produces unique facet joint capsule strain patterns compared with axial rotations. *J Manipulative Physiol Ther*. 2005;28(9):673-687.

15. Cascioli V, Corr P, Till Ag AG. An investigation into the production of intra-articular gas bubbles and increase in joint space in the zygapophyseal joints of the cervical spine in asymptomatic subjects after spinal manipulation. *J Manipulative Physiol Ther*. 2003;26(6):356-364.

16. Cramer GD, Tuck NR, Jr., Knudsen JT, et al. Effects of side-posture positioning and side-posture adjusting on the lumbar zygapophysial joints as evaluated by magnetic resonance imaging: a before and after study with randomization. *J Manipulative Physiol Ther*. 2000;23(6):380-394.

17. Fernandez-de-Las-Penas C, Alonso-Blanco C, Cleland JA, Rodriguez-Blanco C, Alburquerque-Sendin F. Changes in pressure pain thresholds over C5-C6 zygapophyseal joint after a cervicothoracic junction manipulation in healthy subjects. *J Manipulative Physiol Ther*. 2008;31(5):332-337.

18. Pickar JG. Neurophysiological effects of spinal manipulation. *Spine J*. 2002;2(5):357-371.

19. McLain RF. Mechanoreceptor endings in human cervical facet joints. *Spine*. 1994;19(5):495-501.

20. Aprill C, Bogduk N. The prevalence of cervical zygapophyseal joint pain. A first approximation. Spine. 1992;17(7):744-747.

21. Barnsley L, Lord S, Bogduk N. Comparative local anaesthetic blocks in the diagnosis of cervical zygapophysial joint pain. *Pain*. 1993;55(1):99-106.

22. Barnsley L, Bogduk N. Medial branch blocks are specific for the diagnosis of cervical zygapophyseal joint pain. *Reg Anesth*. 1993;18(6):343-350.

23. Coronado RA, Gay CW, Bialosky JE, Carnaby GD, Bishop MD, George SZ. Changes in pain sensitivity following spinal manipulation: a systematic review and meta-analysis. *J Electromyogr Kinesiol*. 2012;22(5):752-767.

24. Wright A. Hypoalgesia post-manipulative therapy: a review of a potential neurophysiological mechanism. *Man Ther*. 1995;1(1):11-16.

25. Ruiz-Saez M, Fernandez-de-las-Penas C, Blanco CR, Martinez-Segura R, Garcia-Leon R. Changes in pressure pain sensitivity in latent myofascial trigger points in the upper trapezius muscle after a cervical spine manipulation in pain-free subjects. *J Manipulative Physiol Ther.* 2007;30(8):578-583.

26. Fernandez-Carnero J, Fernandez-de-las-Penas C, Cleland JA. Immediate hypoalgesic and motor effects after a single cervical spine manipulation in subjects with lateral epicondylalgia. *J Manipulative Physiol Ther.* 2008;31(9):675-681.

27. Haavik-Taylor H, Murphy B. Cervical spine manipulation alters sensorimotor integration: a somatosensory evoked potential study. *Clin Neurophysiol.* 2007;118(2):391-402.

28. Teodorczyk-Injeyan JA, Injeyan HS, Ruegg R. Spinal manipulative therapy reduces inflammatory cytokines but not substance P production in normal subjects. *J Manipulative Physiol Ther.* 2006;29(1):14-21.

29. Degenhardt BF, Darmani NA, Johnson JC, et al. Role of osteopathic manipulative treatment in altering pain biomarkers: a pilot study. *J Am Osteopath Assoc.* 2007;107(9):387-400.

30. Bishop MD, Beneciuk JM, George SZ. Immediate reduction in temporal sensory summation after thoracic spinal manipulation. *Spine J.* 2011;11(5):440-446.

31. Bialosky JE, Bishop MD, Price DD, Robinson ME, George SZ. The mechanisms of manual therapy in the treatment of musculoskeletal pain: a comprehensive model. *Man Ther.* 2009;14(5):531-538.

32. Gensini GF, Conti AA, Conti A. Past and present of "what will please the lord": an updated history of the concept of placebo. *Minerva Med.* 2005;96(2):121-124.

33. Vase L, Riley JL, 3rd, Price DD. A comparison of placebo effects in clinical analgesic trials versus studies of placebo analgesia. *Pain.* 2002;99(3):443-452.

34. Vase L, Petersen GL, Riley JL, 3rd, Price DD. Factors contributing to large analgesic effects in placebo mechanism studies conducted between 2002 and 2007. *Pain.* 2009;145(1-2):36-44.

35. Matre D, Casey KL, Knardahl S. Placebo-induced changes in spinal cord pain processing. *J Neurosci.* 2006;26(2):559-563.

36. Price DD, Craggs J, Verne GN, Perlstein WM, Robinson ME. Placebo analgesia is accompanied by large reductions in pain-related brain activity in irritable bowel syndrome patients. *Pain.* 2007;127(1-2):63-72.

37. Craggs JG, Price DD, Verne GN, Perlstein WM, Robinson MM. Functional brain interactions that serve cognitive-affective processing during pain and placebo analgesia. *NeuroImage.* 2007;38(4):720-729.

38. Sauro MD, Greenberg RP. Endogenous opiates and the placebo effect: a meta-analytic review. *J Psychosom Res.* 2005;58(2):115-120.

39. de la Fuente-Fernandez R, Lidstone S, Stoessl AJ. Placebo effect and dopamine release. *J Neural Transm Suppl.* 2006(70):415-418.

40. Bingel U, Wanigasekera V, Wiech K, et al. The Effect of Treatment Expectation on Drug Efficacy: Imaging the Analgesic Benefit of the Opioid Remifentanil. *Science Translational Medicine.* 2011;3(70):70ra14.

41. Bishop MD, Mintken PE, Bialosky JE, Cleland JA. Patient expectations of benefit from interventions for neck pain and resulting influence on outcomes. *J Orthop Sports Phys Ther.* 2013;43(7):457-465.

42. Puentedura EJ, Flynn T. Combining manual therapy with pain neuroscience education in the treatment of chronic low back pain: A narrative review of the literature. *Physiother Theory Pract.* 2016;32(5):408-414.

43. Louw A, Diener I, Butler DS, Puentedura EJ. The effect of neuroscience education on pain, disability, anxiety, and stress in chronic musculoskeletal pain. *Arch Phys Med Rehabil.* 2011;92(12):2041-2056.

44. Clarke CL, Ryan CG, Martin DJ. Pain neurophysiology education for the management of individuals with chronic low back pain: systematic review and meta-analysis. *Man Ther.* 2011;16(6):544-549.

45. Moseley GL, Nicholas MK, Hodges PW. A randomized controlled trial of intensive neurophysiology education in chronic low back pain. *Clin J Pain.* 2004;20(5):324-330.

46. Moseley L. Combined physiotherapy and education is efficacious for chronic low back pain. *Australian Journal of Physiotherapy.* 2002;48(4):297-302.

47. Moseley L. Unraveling the barriers to reconceptualization of the problem in chronic pain: the actual and perceived ability of patients and health professionals to understand the neurophysiology. *J Pain.* 2003;4(4):184-189.

48. Moseley GL. Joining Forces – Combining Cognition-Targeted Motor Control Training with Group or Individual Pain Physiology Education: A Successful Treatment For Chronic Low Back Pain. *Journal of Manual & Manipulative Therapy.* 2003;11(2):88-94.

49. Moseley GL. Evidence for a direct relationship between cognitive and physical change during an education intervention in people with chronic low back pain. *Eur J Pain*. 2004;8(1):39-45.

50. Moseley GL. Widespread brain activity during an abdominal task markedly reduced after pain physiology education: fMRI evaluation of a single patient with chronic low back pain. *Aust J Physiother*. 2005;51(1):49-52.

51. Tiemann L, May ES, Postorino M, et al. Differential neurophysiological correlates of bottom-up and top-down modulations of pain. *Pain*. 2015;156(2):289-296.

52. Gifford L. Topical Issues in Pain 1. In: Gifford L, ed. *Whiplash: science and management*. Bloomington IN: Author House UK Ltd.; 2013.

53. Colloca CJ, Keller TS, Harrison DE, Moore RJ, Gunzburg R, Harrison DD. Spinal manipulation force and duration affect vertebral movement and neuromuscular responses. *Clin Biomech (Bristol, Avon)*. 2006;21(3):254-262.

54. Hsieh JC, Belfrage M, Stone-Elander S, Hansson P, Ingvar M. Central representation of chronic ongoing neuropathic pain studied by positron emission tomography. *Pain*. 1995;63(2):225-236.

55. Di Blasi Z, Harkness E, Ernst E, Georgiou A, Kleijnen J. Influence of context effects on health outcomes: a systematic review. *Lancet*. 2001;357(9258):757-762.

56. Moseley GL. Why do people with complex regional pain syndrome take longer to recognize their affected hand? *Neurology*. 2004;62(12):2182-2186.

57. Elsig S, Luomajoki H, Sattelmayer M, Taeymans J, Tal-Akabi A, Hilfiker R. Sensorimotor tests, such as movement control and laterality judgment accuracy, in persons with recurrent neck pain and controls. A case-control study. *Man Ther*. 2014;19(6):555-561.

58. Bray H, Moseley GL. Disrupted working body schema of the trunk in people with back pain. *Br J Sports Med*. 2011;45(3):168-173.

59. Bowering KJ, Butler DS, Fulton IJ, Moseley GL. Motor imagery in people with a history of back pain, current back pain, both, or neither. *Clin J Pain*. 2014;30(12):1070-1075.

60. Moseley GL. I can't find it! Distorted body image and tactile dysfunction in patients with chronic back pain. *Pain*. 2008;140(1):239-243.

61. Louw A, Puentedura E. *Therapeutic Neuroscience Education: Teaching patients about pain*. Minneapolis, MN: OPTP; 2013.

62. Moseley GL, Zalucki NM, Wiech K. Tactile discrimination, but not tactile stimulation alone, reduces chronic limb pain. *Pain*. 2008;137(3):600-608.

63. Moseley GL, Wiech K. The effect of tactile discrimination training is enhanced when patients watch the reflected image of their unaffected limb during training. *Pain*. 2009;144(3):314-319.

Chapter 5

Drills and Exercises to Improve Speed and Skills

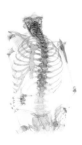

5.1: Chapter Objectives

In this chapter, we present some drills and exercises/activities that we believe will help the practitioner improve their speed and skill in the delivery of thrust joint manipulation. The basic psychomotor skills of thrust joint manipulation techniques can be learned very quickly; however, refinement and skill enhancement requires repetition and practice. We like the analogy of learning to play a musical instrument, let's say the guitar. We can very quickly learn basic chords and strumming techniques, and soon be annoying our family and friends with our renditions of contemporary songs. But if we aspire to play the guitar like a virtuoso (e.g. Eric Clapton), then we should expect that it will take lots and lots of practice. Musicians refine and improve their skill through the use of musical scales and musical drills, and so can we with thrust joint manipulation techniques. The skills that any seasoned manual therapy practitioner possesses in the delivery of thrust joint manipulation will have been learned and practiced for many years. As seasoned manual therapy practitioners, we have learned and shared various drills to enhance skill, and it is these drills that we wish we had been taught all those years ago when we first began learning thrust joint techniques. Clinical experience leads us to believe that they enhance skill acquisition and will assist with the acquisition of expertise at a much faster rate.

5.2: Are Highly Developed Skills Necessary?

The available research literature appears to suggest that manipulative therapists cannot be level-specific with their techniques. Ross et al[1] completed an evaluation study in which they used accelerometers to locate the joints that produced an audible sound in response to manipulation (i.e. cavitation) so that the accuracy and specificity of the manipulative technique could be assessed. Sixty-four asymptomatic subjects had their thoracic and lumbar spines manipulated by 28 clinicians while they were 'wired' with these accelerometers. Their results found that when clinicians indicated which level of the thoracic or lumbar spine they were targeting with their technique, they were only accurate in the lumbar spine 46 percent of the time (57/124) and 54 percent of the time (29/54) in the thoracic spine. However, it is important to note that the technique was declared accurate if a cavitation occurred at the designated spinal joint, and the researchers found that most of the techniques produced multiple cavitations. Therefore, if at least one cavitation emanated from the targeted joints, the technique was declared accurate. Furthermore, the clinicians participating in the study were all Canadian chiropractors who had a range of experience of one to 43 years. A critical review of this particular study leads us to conclude that Canadian chiropractors are not terribly accurate with their manipulative techniques, and really, that is all that should be concluded from this study. Furthermore, if most of the techniques generated multiple cavitations (as indicated in the study) then it would appear that the clinicians used more generalized (let's get as many of the joints to cavitate) rather than more localized techniques (let's take the time to set things up correctly and apply minimal force to achieve a single cavitation).

Another study by Bolton et al[2] used skin mounted microphones along the articular pillars at the C2 level to determine which side of the cervical spine produced the cavitation during a cervical spine manipulation. In this study, a single practitioner provided either 'rotation' or 'lateral flexion' manipulative techniques to 22 asymptomatic subjects. The subjects were asked to provide their perception of the location of the cavitation sounds they experienced. Interestingly, the researchers found that with 'rotation' thrusts, cavitation was more likely to occur on the contralateral side to the applicator (p=0.02). With 'lateral flexion' thrusts, there was no significant correlation between the side of cavitation and the side of the applicator (p=0.350). This means that when performing a rotation technique to the left, with the manipulative applicator on the right articular pillar, this single practitioner was more likely to achieve a cavitation on the left articular pillar instead of the right. And, with lateral flexion to the left, either side was just as likely to cavitate. Finally, there was limited agreement between subject perceptions and the actual side of cavitation (kappa = 0.40), meaning that the subjects were not able to tell which side had been manipulated. Again, a critical review of this study should lead us to conclude (quite simply) that the single practitioner (Osteopath in New Zealand) in this study was not particularly accurate or specific with his manipulative thrust techniques.

It has been suggested, based on these two studies, that clinicians cannot be accurate and level-specific in the delivery of their manipulative techniques. Furthermore, recent studies have found that the audible cavitation associated with spinal manipulation in the low back may not be necessary to achieve improvement in outcomes.[3,4] These studies were secondary analyses of data from clinical prediction rule development and validation studies. Clinicians recorded whether an audible cavitation was heard by either the patient with low back pain or the therapist. The outcome was assessed with the 11-point numeric pain rating scale, the Oswestry Disability Questionnaire and measurement of lumbopelvic flexion range of motion. Repeated measures analyses of variance (ANOVA) were used to examine whether the achievement of a cavitation resulted in improved outcome. Although cavitation was perceived in 84 percent of patients, no differences were detected at any follow-up period in the level of pain, disability or lumbopelvic range of motion based on whether a cavitation was achieved (p>0.05). This led the authors to suggest that a perceived audible cavitation may not relate to improved outcomes from thrust joint manipulation for patients with non-radicular low back pain.

Similarly, a study by Haas et al[5] reported on the response of patients with neck pain who received thrust joint manipulation to either a randomly assigned level or a level selected based on end-play assessment. The authors found that both groups achieved equally significant reduction in neck pain and stiffness, with no apparent advantage in attempting to target the intervention to specifically identified spinal segments.

These research findings, suggesting that clinicians cannot be accurate nor level-specific when providing thrust joint manipulation, should not reduce the need for continued emphasis on developing expert patient-handling skills in manual therapy. Some in the field of physical therapy have recommended a greater emphasis on evidence-based decision making and the development of hands-on skills that can be performed proficiently. There have been calls for therapists to 'move it and move on.'[6] While we agree that there should be an emphasis on evidence-based decision making, we would argue that there should also be an incentive to develop excellent hands-on skills so that they can be performed, not just proficiently, but safely, effectively and skillfully.

Transient side effects are very common following thrust joint manipulation.[7-9] A prospective survey of side effects from spinal manipulation among physical therapists, chiropractors, and osteopaths in Belgium found that 238/465 (60.9 percent) of patients experienced at least one side effect.[7] Another survey study involving 1,058 patients treated with spinal manipulation by chiropractors in Norway reported that 55 percent of patients reported at least one side effect, which was rated as mild to moderate in 85 percent of these individuals.[8] Similarly, a survey of 625 patients treated with 1,858 thrust joint manipulation interventions found that 44 percent reported at least one side effect.[9] It is our belief that these transient side effects following thrust joint manipulation may be the result of poorly delivered thrust techniques. By poorly delivered, we mean excessive force production, and/or excessive amplitude of movement, and/or insufficient speed of technique. We base this belief on our combined 80 years of clinical experience using thrust joint manipulation techniques. What we have noticed over the years, is that as our skills have improved, we have become more refined in the performance of thrust joint techniques, our patients have reported experiencing less frequent side effects. Ultimately, it should all be about patient comfort and achieving the best outcome for the patient with the least discomfort. It must be an advantage when the clinician is more than just proficient, and he or she is highly skilled and precise in the delivery of such techniques.

5.3: Amplitude Drills

Amplitude drills are devised to develop the correct amount of pressure and distance to engaging the barrier without overshooting it. These drills should teach you to engage the barrier without causing damage to the joint from loss of control and too much force. They will also teach you to use the larger muscles to control the amplitude.

Plinth drill: Stand over a treatment plinth and place one hand over the other then do a rapid compression into the plinth (Figure 5.3a). Go to the "end feel" by locating the point where you have compressed all of the cushioning and can feel the wooden base of the plinth, and then go no farther.

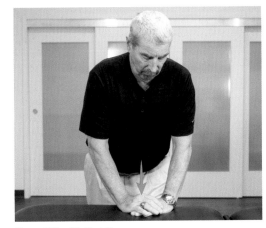

Figure 5.3a: Plinth drill.

Keeping the elbows slightly bent, find the end feel and apply a quick thrust into the table keeping one foot back. Your elbows should extend quickly but not fully as you make quick contractions of your pectorals.

Karate punch drill: Perform a karate punch into a soft surface but hold up just before going any deeper than a superficial indent. A piece of paper or pillow will serve this purpose (Figure 5.3b). This can also be done into the plinth. The idea is to hit the surface rapidly (speed) but lightly (not forcefully) by stopping at the point of contact with the paper or pillow.

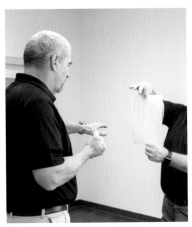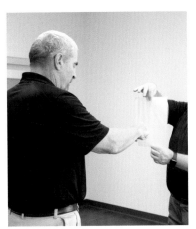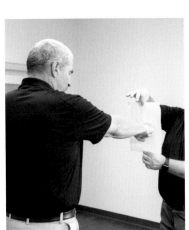

Figure 5.3b: Karate punch drill.

Bubble wrap manipulation: For this drill, you should use bubble wrap that has the softer, larger bubbles. This can be purchased at any office supply store. Mark a single bubble and attempt to pop it using specific manipulation without breaking the surrounding bubbles (Figure 5.3c). This can be achieved with the pisiform grip, a single digit or both thumbs.

Lateral shoulder push: This drill can be used by the clinician to learn how to control amplitude and speed with thrust manipulations. Two people are required for this drill. The clinician should stand to the side of his/her partner, and place their thrusting hand over the lateral deltoid muscles, keeping his/her elbow slightly flexed (Figure 5.3d). The clinician should have the foot on the side of the thrusting hand placed back. The clinician should gently push into the deltoids a few times to test the barrier (i.e. the point at which their partner will be moved). The clinician then applies a short, quick impulse to the lateral deltoids of the partner. This should only involve slight movement of the person's shoulder.

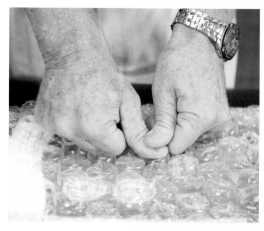

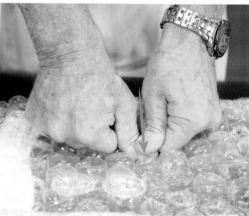

Figure 5.3c: Bubble wrap manipulation.

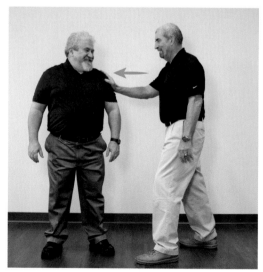

Figure 5.3d: Lateral shoulder push.

5.4: Large Muscle Groups

Large muscle group drill: (adapted from martial arts drills) Use the metacarpophalangeal (MCP) joint of index finger and apply a rapid impulse into the palm of the opposite hand (Figure 5.4a). Repeat this several times and then switch hands. With this drill, vary the amplitude of the thrust into the opposite hand by focusing on use of the large muscles (i.e. pectorals, biceps and lats).

Large muscle drill for use of the shoulder in lumbar manipulation: This drill helps the therapist time the direction of the thrusting arm and shoulder when performing a lumbar manipulation. Stand with the elbow flexed to 90 degrees and first rapidly depresses their shoulder. Then forcefully contract the shoulder into extension with rapid but short amplitude. Then combine the two movements together producing combination of rapid shoulder depression and extension simultaneously (Figure 5.4b). Finally, add a drop to the back foot on that side while performing the same motion in the shoulder. Make sure the spine is straight when performing this movement.

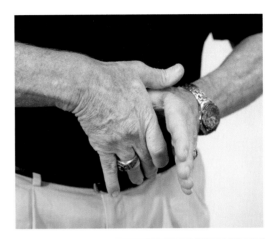

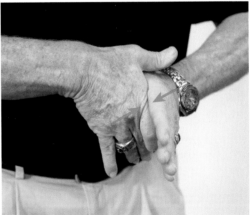

Figure 5.4a: Large muscle group drill.

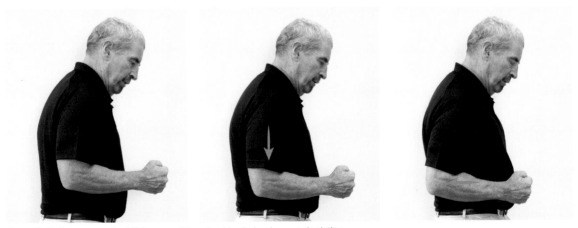

Figure 5.4b: Large muscle drill for use of the shoulder in lumbar manipulation.

5.5: Coordination, Core, Stance and Response to Motion Drills

These drills help train the therapist to use their trunk/core to apply the thrust in combination with the thrusting arm. These will also allow the therapist to appreciate movement in space through the arms and trunk.

Ball drill: Stand facing a partner with one foot forward and place a 10" ball sandwiched between outstretch hands. This ball can be purchased at any toy store. Take turns pushing and pulling without dropping the ball to develop coordination and response to motion (Figure 5.5a).

Hand motion drill: Find a partner and stand facing each other. Extend the arm slightly and place the palm of the hand against the palm of the hand of your partner. One of you will be the mover and the other will be the follower. Take turns moving in different planes, directions, and speeds while trying to keep the hands in contact with minimum pressure (Figure 5.5b). The follower will try to respond to the movements of the mover to develop a sense of a barrier. To make it more challenging, place the back of the hand against the back of your partner's hand and perform the same motions.

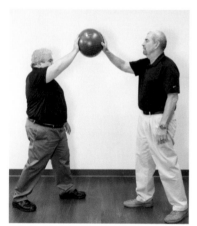 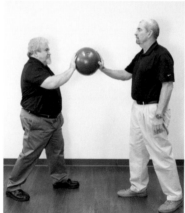 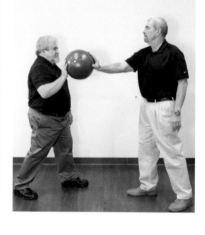

Figure 5.5a: Ball drill.

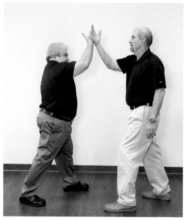 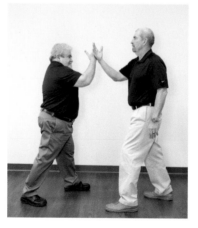 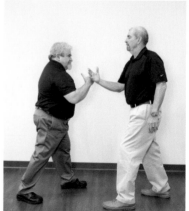

Figure 5.5b: Hand motion drill.

Hand shake: Stand facing your partner with legs parallel to each other and reach out to gently shake their hand. Then place one leg back. With the hand on the side of back leg, shake your partner's hand again (Figure 5.5c). Feel the difference in the stability through the hand and arm. (Courtesy of Laurie Hartman)

Core and stance drill: Pair off with each person facing each other. One will stand with the feet parallel while the other will stand with one foot back. Each person will alternately (while grasping each other's hands) pull each

partner toward each other (Figure 5.5d). The person with the foot back will be able to pull that person with their feet parallel toward them off balance. The person with the foot back should be able to maintain their stance when pulled by their partner. When adding core stabilization by tightening the core it is almost impossible to pull this person off balance. The parallel leg stance will not provide the stability that the staggered stance will. This illustrates the importance of stance and stability in performing thrusts. (Courtesy of Laurie Hartman)

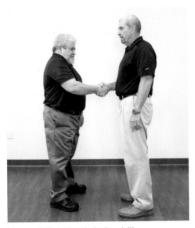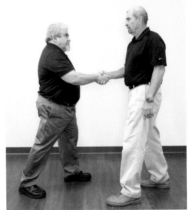

Figure 5.5c: Hand shake drill.

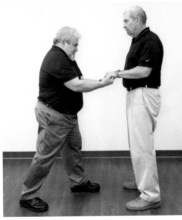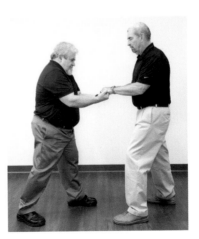

Figure 5.5d: Core and stance drill.

5.6: Speed Drills

These drills should help develop speed by engaging the larger proximal muscles needed to do this. Speed is absolutely necessary to break through tissue resistance.

Toilet paper pull: Rapidly pull one sheet of toilet paper off without unraveling the roll. Try with two hands and then one (Figure 5.6a). Try tearing off more than more than one sheet at a time.

Dollar bill drop: Hold crisp dollar bill just above your partner's opened thumb and index finger. Let it drop suddenly between your partner's opened thumb and index finger while they attempt to grab it (Figure 5.6b). This drill can be made more challenging by widening the distance between the thumb and index finger. It takes anticipation and speed with the thumb and index finger to catch the dollar bill before it falls past their grip. Once you have tried this a few times, have your partner hold two palms apart and do the same thing. They should be much more successful at catching the bill with two palms, and this helps illustrate that use of the larger muscle groups improves reaction and speed.

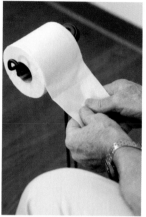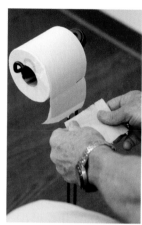

Figure 5.6a: Toilet paper pull.

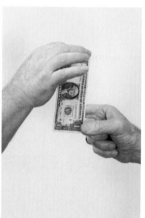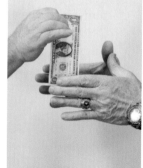

Figure 5.6b: Dollar bill drop.

Coin grab: Place a coin (a quarter works best) in the open palm. Have your partner place their open palm next to yours and then try to grab the coin out of your hand before you close it (Figure 5.6c). Trade places and try to grab the coin from your partner's hand before they close their palm. To make it more challenging, reach from below the other person's hand and try to grab the coin. Try this with larger coins at first and progress to smaller ones as you improve.

Pringles can drill: Fill an empty Pringles can with dried beans or rice and seal it. Use the smallest and next to the smallest cans. With both hands, grab one end and snap it, driving the contents to the other end of the can. Do this as quickly as possible to create a single noise as the contents snap from one end of the can to the other (Figure 5.6d). You can also grab the can on either end and quickly turn it from side to side, simulating a cervical manipulation, forcing the contents to one end of the can. Try this all to the right and then to the left. (Courtesy of Elaine and Paul Lonneman)

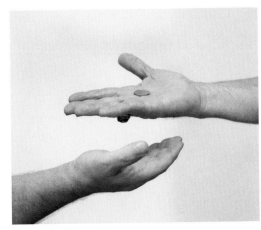

Figure 5.6c: Coin grab.

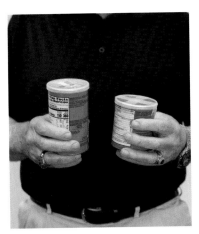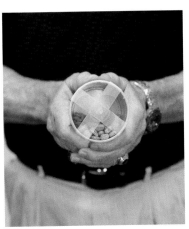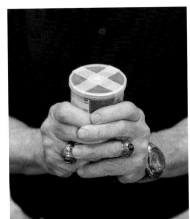

Figure 5.6d: Pringles can drill.

Banana break: Get a banana and grab it with both hands close together. Try to break it cleanly into two pieces without splattering the ends (Figure 5.6e). This requires speed and is easier with unripe bananas but is much harder with ones that are a little more soft and ripe. Try it with the hands further apart. (Courtesy of Laurie McLaughlin)

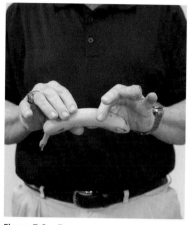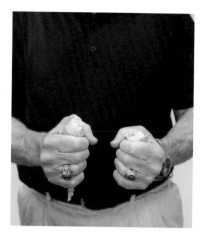

Figure 5.6e: Banana break.

Egg drill: Place a towel on the table, and then within the towel place a raw egg. Fold the towel over the egg, and then place both hands over the egg and thrust the egg into the table without breaking it (Figure 5.6f). Do this by cupping your bottom hand. To make it more challenging, place a pillow over the egg and try to find the egg. Then perform the same thrust.

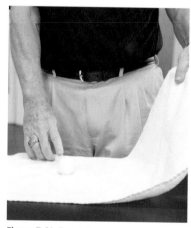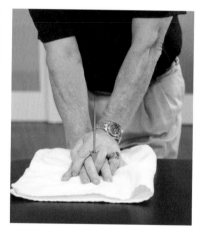

Figure 5.6f: Egg drill.

Flick: Hold an empty aluminum soda can, as if to twist it in half in its middle. Twist quickly with both hands without denting the can (Figure 5.6g). This drill helps you practice rapid pronation/supination motions with the hands.

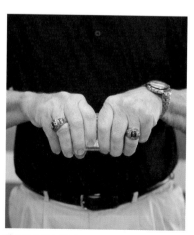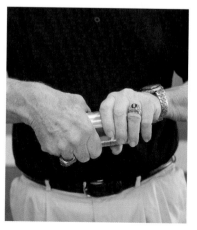

Figure 5.6g: Flick.

5.7: Leg Drops, Pivot and Weight Shifting Drills

These drills are designed to develop use of the legs in applying the thrust and encouraging the dropping back onto the back leg when applying techniques like lumbar thrusts. These additional drills should also help you use your body to move the patient to the barrier and will allow you to feel the movement better using the more plentiful proprioceptors of your trunk.

Heel drops: Stand with one leg in front and the other behind, and have the heel of the back leg off the ground. Relax your body, then, as rapidly as possible, drop your weight onto the rear heel (Figure 5.7a). Speed not force is the key here.

Knee buckles: Stand in a relaxed manner, then allow your knees to buckle rapidly under control, with a short amplitude drop (Figure 5.7b).

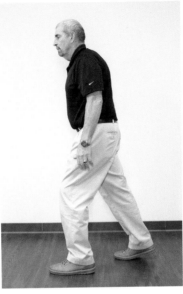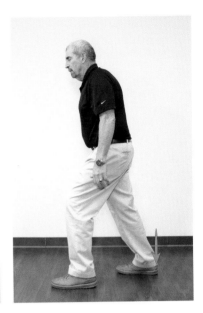

Figure 5.7a: Heel drops.

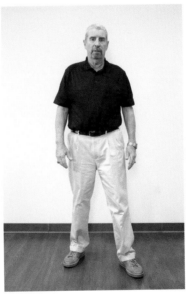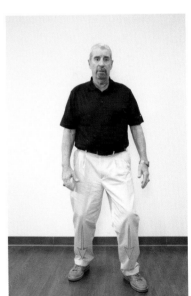

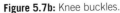
Figure 5.7b: Knee buckles.

Weight shift drills: These drills will help prepare you to move your body when evaluating motion and applying techniques and using your core. Hands and arms should remain still while your body moves, shifting weight from side to side, bending one knee then the other (Figure 5.7c). Then place feet apart and move your butt from side to side.

Pivot drills: Stand with one foot back and the other forward, then pivot on both feet to turn completely to the left or right (Figure 5.7d). This drill should help you align yourself correctly to the patient, and to the direction of the thrust.

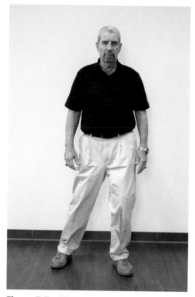 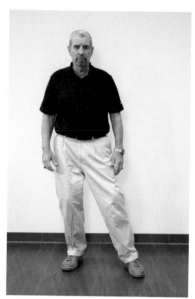

Figure 5.7c: Weight shift drills.

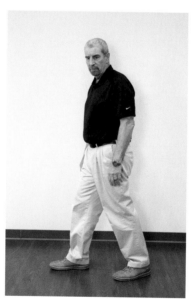 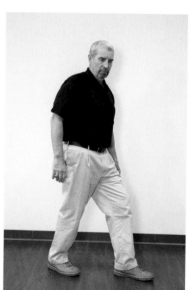

Figure 5.7d: Pivot drills.

5.8: Enhancing Palpation Skills and Segment Location

These are a few drills that should help the therapist to enhance their palpation skills. They are designed to allow for greater appreciation and localization of the manipulative barrier.

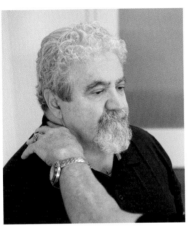 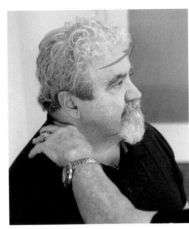 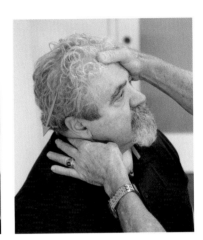

Figure 5.8a: Palpation of C spine to get the feel of the barrier.

Palpation of C spine to get the feel of the barrier: In the standing or sitting position, pair off with a partner. Place the lateral or radial border of your index finger with a very light touch onto the lamina of a mid-cervical segment (Figure 5.8a). Keeping the finger in place, have your partner rotate the neck away until you feel movement under your finger. It is a sense of fullness as you are feeling lamina through a lot of tissue. Continue by having them side-bend to the same side over your finger until you begin to feel the fullness over your finger. Then have your partner extend the neck until movement is felt at that segment. Then, holding your partner's head in this position, check the primary lever of rotation away and you should find that you have engaged the barrier.

Hand grasp palpation drill: This drill is designed to give the therapist a sense of how much pressure to apply when handling the spine. It is particularly helpful in palpating or placing the hands on the cervical spine. Too often, palpation is performed too deeply and firmly to be able to appreciate the tissue you are trying to target. Partner up and grasp each other's hands. One person at a time, slowly increase the grip pressure to your partner's hand. Apply only enough force such that there is minimal muscle contraction in the forearm, yet apply enough contact to appreciate the hand tissues of your partner. Palpate the muscles with your opposite hand or have your partner do it (Figure 5.8b). (Courtesy of Joe Farrell)

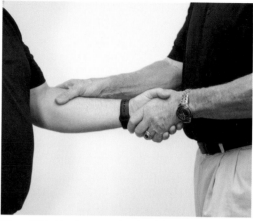

Figure 5.8b: Hand grasp palpation drill.

Towel drill for localization:
Grab a hand towel or small bath towel by both ends and twist it on itself to engage an end feel of sorts, but not to the point where the towel starts to bend from being too tight. Then you can add side-bending with it to further engage the barrier and further add tension by applying traction or translating to test the tension or barrier you have created (Figure 5.8c). (Courtesy of Elaine and Paul Lonneman)

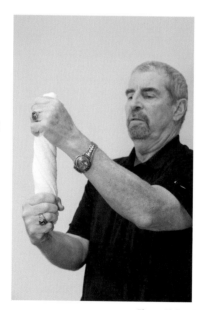
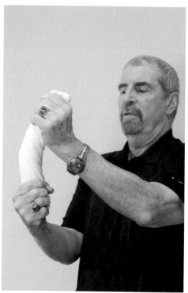

Figure 5.8c: Towel drill for localization.

5.9: Key Points from Chapter 5

- Thrust joint manipulation to the spine, like any other psychomotor skill, requires sufficient practice to advance from proficiency to mastery.

- Although there is evidence to suggest that *some* clinicians are not accurate and level-specific when performing spinal manipulation, there is no evidence to suggest it applies to *all* clinicians.

- Mastery of thrust joint manipulation skills can be achieved through the performance of appropriate training drills and repetitive practice.

- In this chapter, we presented some drills we have used to advance our skills by focusing on the development and control of amplitude, force generation and speed.

- It is also important for the clinician to work on improving control of their posture and use of the large muscle groups to ensure technique refinement.

Chapter 5 References

1. Ross JK, Bereznick DE, McGill SM. Determining cavitation location during lumbar and thoracic spinal manipulation: is spinal manipulation accurate and specific? *Spine (Phila Pa 1976)*. 2004;29(13):1452-1457.

2. Bolton A, Moran RW, Standen C. An investigation into the side of joint cavitation associated with cervical spine manipulation. *International Journal of Osteopathic Medicine*. 2007;10(4):88-96.

3. Flynn TW, Fritz JM, Wainner RS, Whitman JM. The audible pop is not necessary for successful spinal high-velocity thrust manipulation in individuals with low back pain. *Arch Phys Med Rehabil*. 2003;84(7):1057-1060.

4. Flynn TW, Childs JD, Fritz JM. The audible pop from high-velocity thrust manipulation and outcome in individuals with low back pain. *J Manipulative Physiol Ther*. 2006;29(1):40-45.

5. Haas M, Groupp E, Panzer D, Partna L, Lumsden S, Aickin M. Efficacy of cervical endplay assessment as an indicator for spinal manipulation. *Spine (Phila Pa 1976)*. 2003;28(11):1091-1096; discussion 1096.

6. Flynn TW. Move It and Move On. *Journal of Orthopaedic & Sports Physical Therapy*. 2002;32(5):192-193.

7. Cagnie B, Vinck E, Beernaert A, Cambier D. How common are side effects of spinal manipulation and can these side effects be predicted? *Man Ther*. 2004;9(3):151-156.

8. Senstad O, Leboeuf-Yde C, Borchgrevink C. Frequency and characteristics of side effects of spinal manipulative therapy. *Spine (Phila Pa 1976)*. 1997;22(4):435-440; discussion 440-431.

9. Leboeuf-Yde C, Hennius B, Rudberg E, Leufvenmark P, Thunman M. Side effects of chiropractic treatment: a prospective study. J *Manipulative Physiol Ther*. 1997;20(8):511-515.

Chapter 6

Physical Tests Prior to Administering Thrust Joint Manipulation Techniques to the Spine

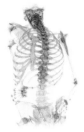

6.1: Chapter Objectives

This chapter will describe the pre-manipulative tests that we recommend be done prior to administering specific thrust joint manipulative techniques. Obviously, there are many other tests that can be included. It is not our intention to be all-inclusive with respect to differential diagnosis and treatment. This book is geared to the demonstration and practical application of thrust joint technique. The tests we recommend are ones that we would use prior to specific manipulation, once "red" and "yellow" flags have been ruled out. There are routine tests that you should perform every time you assess the spine. The other tests specific to areas of the spine, such as the modified Sharp-Purser test, may be considered under the heading of "special" tests. Not all of the tests outlined here may be mentioned in the technique descriptions as suggested tests. All of the tests do not have to be performed unless the patient history dictates they are needed.

We will base our discussion on evidence whenever possible, and present statistical data regarding each test's intra- and interrater reliability and validity (where it is available). However, where no evidence is available, we will base our discussion on our combined clinical experience and hope to present a variety of reasonably reliable tests from which the clinician may choose.

6.2: The Routine Tests

6.2.1: The Pre-Manipulative Hold

With all of the thrust techniques, we would recommend a pre-manipulative hold prior to applying the thrust. In this case, the patient is placed into the position in which they would receive the thrust, and it would be held there for eight to 10 seconds (Figure 6.2.1a). The idea of a pre-manipulative hold is that, in this sustained position, the presence of pain or a more severe adverse reaction to this position would preclude the clinician from going ahead with the thrust joint manipulation.

This pre-manipulative hold can be done for all spinal regions, not just the cervical spine. It should not be confused with the cervical rotation component of the vertebrobasilar insufficiency test where the patient's cervical spine is taken to end range rotation and held there for 10 to 15 seconds.[1,2] We are not aware of any research on the reliability and diagnostic utility of the pre-manipulative hold.

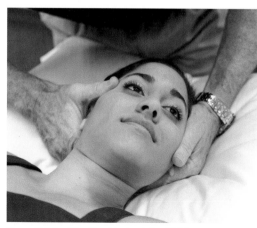

Figure 6.2.1a: The Pre-Manipulative Hold.

6.2.2: AROM and Passive Physiological Intervertebral Motion (PPIVMs)

Testing active motion testing for the spine has been shown to have good inter-examiner reliability, with intraclass correlation coefficients (ICC) values exceeding .75, as long as some kind of measuring device is used.[3-6] Assessing active range of motion via visual estimation is less reliable.[7] In clinical practice, the ease of motion and reports of pain reproduction or aggravation with active motion yield greater information than the specific range in degrees.

Passive physiological intervertebral motion testing for the spine is found to be less reliable. Smedmark et al[8] reported Kappa values ranging from 0.28 to 0.43 for the cervical spine. Brismee et al[9] reported Kappa values ranging from 0.27 to 0.65 for the mid-thoracic spine. And Keating et al[10] reported Kappa values ranging from -0.03 to 0.23 for the lumbar spine. However, again, the ease of motion and pain response during that motion can provide helpful information for the clinician as they work through their clinical reasoning processes. We therefore consider these tests as a necessary part of the assessment of any spinal joint prior to considering manipulation.

6.2.3: Passive Accessory Intervertebral Motions (PAIVMs)

Passive accessory intervertebral motions (PAIVMs) refer to spinal motion assessment techniques developed by Geoff Maitland. PAIVMs are used to test the accessory motions such as glide and translation of the intervertebral joint, and they can be used to assess the relationships between pain, spasm and resistance through joint palpation.

In a landmark study by Matyas and Bach,[11] it was found that palpation for position or resistance had rather poor reliability (Kappa values ranging from 0.01 to 0.46) but palpation for pain response (pain onset or P1) was significantly better (Kappa values ranging from 0.62 to 0.99). As a result, many contemporary clinicians will use PAIVMs with subjective pain responses from their patients to localize spinal motion segments that may be appropriate targets of manual treatment. Phillips and Twomey[12] reported that sensitivity in detecting the symptomatic lumbar segmental level was greater with verbal versus non-verbal subject responses (94 percent vs 53 percent). They concluded that a manual therapist's manual examination, when accompanied by a verbal subject response, is highly accurate in detecting the lumbar segmental level responsible for a subject's complaint.[12] Piva et al[13] reported similar findings for the cervical spine, in that, as long as PAIVMs were assessed as hypomobile or normal and subject response was considered, accuracy in detecting a symptomatic segmental level was high.

6.2.4: Palpation for Pain and Position

These particular evaluation tools are also a necessary staple in the assessment toolbox to be used prior to manipulating the spine. Palpation of painful structures can have excellent reliability where the patient has an acute or sub-acute condition. Localizing painful structures in patients with chronic or widespread pain is another matter. Structures that may be palpated would include bone, ligament, and muscle in the spine.

Palpation for position of the spinal zygapophyseal joints (facets) and the intervertebral spaces has been shown to be less reliable, especially in the absence of subject response.[11-13] However, many clinicians continue to use this palpation as part of their reasoning strategy (Figure 6.2.4a). In a recent survey of 336 Dutch manual therapists, researchers found that respondents believed that motion and position palpation tests were important for treatment decisions and were confident in their conclusions drawn from it.[14]

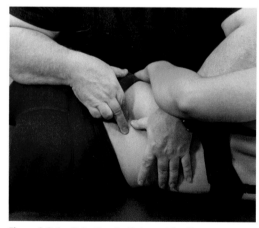

Figure 6.2.4a: Palpation for Pain and Position.

6.2.5: Spring Testing and PA Testing

Spring testing and PA testing are essentially the same thing. Some manual therapy clinicians will prefer to call the use of a pisiform contact as Spring testing, and use of the thumbs as PA testing, but essentially, both tests can be used to assess motion and pain response over any segment of the spine. For the thoracic and lumbar motion segments, the pisiform contact is more comfortable for both the clinician and the patient. By overlapping the hands and using the pisiform of the bottom hand to contact the spinous process, that bottom hand resting on the spine does no work. The top hand does most of the work by pushing into the bottom hand. It is important when performing this test that the clinician stay as upright as possible with the arms pretty straight at the elbows. It is most comfortable on clinician and patient alike when clinicians use their body to lean into the patient. The clinician is able to feel more (gauge the stiffness of the motion segment as hypomobile, normal or hypermobile) through recruiting the large proprioceptors of the body.

PA testing using the thumb pads can also be used in the entire spine (Figure 6.2.5a). It, like the spring test, is more successful and gentler on the patient when the clinician leans into the segment through their thumbs. There are variations to doing PA testing with the thumbs. They can be placed one on top of the other, or facing nail bed to nail bed. It is probably more comfortable, in the authors' experience, to superimpose one thumb over the other, especially when stronger grades of motion are required.

As already discussed, reliability of palpation is generally higher when patient response is taken into account. Spring and PA testing is also a psychomotor skill that the clinician can develop into a valuable clinical assessment and treatment tool with practice (Figure 6.2.5a). The late Geoffrey Maitland[15] pioneered the use of this type of passive mobilization for pain modulation, and refined this skill with great precision. His models for practice and his descriptions of examination and treatment techniques continue to be standard methodology for many manual therapy clinicians and researchers.

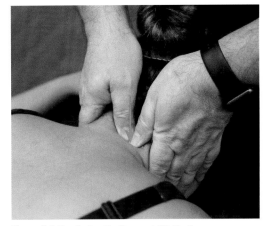

Figure 6.2.5a: Spring Testing and PA Testing.

6.3: Special Tests

6.3.1: The Friedman-Johnston Tap Test

Renowned British osteopath Laurie Hartman first introduced this test to the authors many years ago. The test was developed by William Johnston DO, from East Lansing over 30 years ago.[16] Although there appears to be limited research on this test, the published studies that we found seem to indicate this test has a better than average reliability.[16-19] The test itself involves tapping quickly along the spine (Figure 6.3.1a), and the contact points of the evaluator's hand can be the index and ring finger on the patient's transverse processes at each level. It is important that the therapist keep the wrist limp enough so that their hand literally bounces off the spine.

The therapist is looking for changes in tympani or resonance from one segment to another. The sound and feel under an affected segment tapped is noted to have a different pitch and 'stiffness' than the adjacent ones. Finding a positive responsive level does not indicate what kind of dysfunction might be present; simply that something is going on at that level. If the therapist continues tapping over the responsive segment, they will often note

a noxious response to it from the patient. Dr. Hartman, in personal dialogue with the authors, described the difference in testing in prone and seated: "The main difference is that the postural muscles are not working when the patient is prone, so any dysfunction will be less evident than when they are sitting. If it is more evident, this means that we can get them better with manual therapy usually with a manipulation. If it disappears completely, then we have to get the posture sorted out, which will take longer."[20]

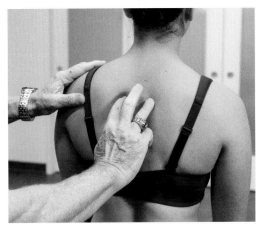

Figure 6.3.1a: The Friedman-Johnston Tap Test.

6.3.2: Thoracic Inspiration Test with Flexion and Extension

The patient is in the seated position on a treatment table without back support. They are first passively flexed and asked to take in a deep breath. Then they are placed in extension and asked to take another deep breath (Figure 6.3.2a). If they report pain only in extension, it is more suggestive of a facet joint problem. Inspiration causes additional extension motion at the facet joints. It therefore acts like an overpressure when the facets are already closed down in the extended position. If the patient reports pain with inspiration in both positions, then it is thought that the problem could be coming from the ribs.

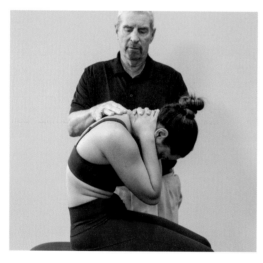

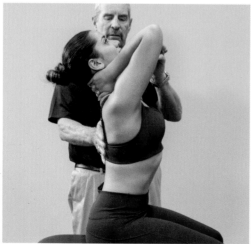

Figure 6.3.2a: Thoracic Inspiration Test with Flexion and Extension.

6.3.3: Sacroiliac (SI) Joint Tests

Several studies by Mark Laslett[21-23] and co-authors[24-27], as well as work conducted by Van der Wurff and colleagues[28-34] have demonstrated that there probably isn't one perfect sacroiliac (SI) joint provocative test that we can perform to definitively diagnose SI joint pain or dysfunction. The combination of these studies leaves us with six pain provocation tests that can be used to rule in or rule out SI joint dysfunction. These are Gaenslen's test (Left and Right), distraction, compression, thigh thrust, and sacral thrust. Laslett[23] reported that the accuracy of detecting SI joint dysfunction is increased when at least three of the six tests are positive. Three or more positive pain provocation SI joint tests have sensitivity and specificity of 91 percent and 78 percent, respectively.[23] Specificity of three or more positive tests increases to 87 percent in patients whose symptoms cannot be made to move toward the spinal midline, i.e., centralize.

Kokmeyer et al[32] examined the interrater reliability of multi-test scores by using a regimen of five commonly used SI pain provocation tests and reported a weighted kappa of 0.70 (95 percent CI = 0.45 - 0.95) indicating good to excellent reliability. Van der Wurff et al[31] found that if at least three out the five tests were positive, there was 85 percent sensitivity and 79 percent specificity for detecting the SI joint as the source of pain. Essentially, if all five tests are negative, one can likely look at structures other that the SI joint. Kokmeyer et al[32], additionally agreed with Laslett[23] and Van der Wurff[31], but found that a positive thigh thrust was good enough to detect the presence of an SI joint dysfunction.

6.3.4: Fortin's Finger Test

Fortin described this test in 1991 as a simple diagnostic aid to clinicians to consider SI joint dysfunction.[35,36] The patient is asked to point to the region of their pain with one finger (Figure 6.3.4a). A positive sign was noted if the patient could: a) localize their pain with one finger; b) the area was immediately inferomedial to the PSIS within one cm; and c) the patient consistently pointed to the same area over at least two trials. This is one of the few SI joint tests that is highly sensitive but has low specificity.[37] This is essentially a test of exclusion, in that if the test is negative, the condition (SI joint problem) can be ruled out.

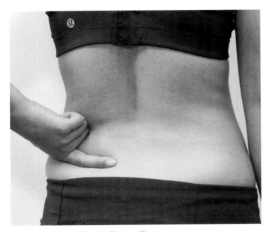

Figure 6.3.4a: Fortin's Finger Test.

6.3.5: Gaenslen's Test

Also known as Gaenslen's maneuver, this is considered an SI joint provocation test. It was first described in 1927 by Frederick Julius Gaenslen.[38] The patient is placed on a table with one leg over the side, and is asked to pull their other knee to the chest. The clinician then applies overpressure to the anterior thigh of the leg hanging off the table while pushing the patient's opposite knee further into their chest (Figure 6.3.5a). A positive response is pain in the SI joint on that side. The test is then performed on the other side and results are compared.

6.3.6: Sacral Compression Test

This test is performed with the patient in a side-lying position. The clinician stands behind the patient with both hands applying a firm downward pressure through the anterior portion of the ilium, compressing the SI joint (Figure 6.3.6a). A positive test is a reproduction of the patient's familiar pain in the SI joint.

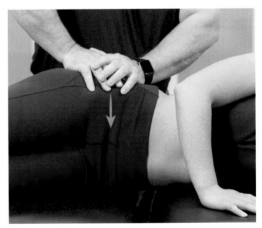

Figure 6.3.6a: Sacral Compression Test.

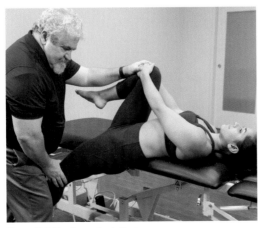

Figure 6.3.5a: Gaenslen's Test.

6.3.7: ASIS Distraction Test

The patient is placed in supine on the table. The clinician places their palms over both ASISs, and applies pressure to spread the ASISs (Figure 6.3.7a). A positive test is a reproduction of the patient's familiar pain in either SI joint.

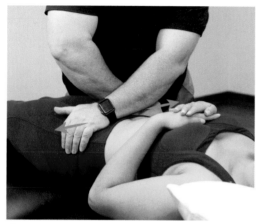

Figure 6.3.7a: ASIS Distraction Test.

6.3.8: Sacral thrust

The patient is placed in prone on the table, and asked to relax. The clinician applies an anterior pressure through the sacrum (Figure 6.3.8a). A positive test is reproduction or aggravation of the patient's familiar pain.

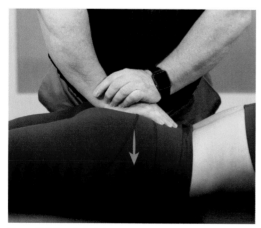

Figure 6.3.8a: Sacral thrust.

6.3.9: Thigh Thrust/Femoral Shear Test

The patient is placed supine on the table. The clinician reaches across the table to the opposite leg, and then passively flexes that knee and hip to 90 degrees and rolls the pelvis toward them. This allows the clinician to place their hand under the patient's sacrum. The clinician then applies a posterior shearing force to the SI joint through the femur (Figure 6.3.9a). It is important to avoid excessive hip adduction during the test as it can provoke hip pain. The clinician can hold the pressure for 30 seconds or can oscillate into the sacrum in attempt to provoke the patient's familiar pain.

According to Laslett et al,[25] two out of four provocation tests (distraction, compression, thigh thrust and sacral thrust) have sensitivity of 0.88 and specificity of 0.78. Positive likelihood ratio (+LR) of 4.00 and negative likelihood ratio (-LR) of 0.16 for SI joint pathology. Alternatively, three out of all six provocation tests (adding in R and L Gaenslen's) have sensitivity of 0.94 and specificity of 0.78. +LR of 4.29 and -LR of 0.80 for SI joint pathology.

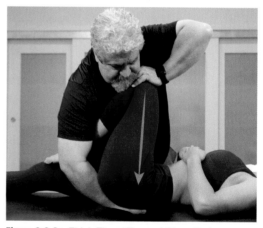

Figure 6.3.9a: Thigh Thrust/Femoral Shear Test.

6.4: Cervical Tests

There are many tests that purport to mechanically stress the upper cervical spine ligaments and identify ligament instability or deficiency. Cook et al[39] stated that clinically relevant cervical spine instability is difficult to diagnose, involves subtle clinical features, and few valid, reliable clinical tests exist to aid in differential diagnosis. Numerous clinical tests for cervical spine instability are currently in use in clinical practice, and most are intended to assess the integrity of the alar and transverse ligaments. However, most of these tests have not been validated in patients with neck pain, and the level of reliability of the tests varies significantly.[39-41] Most clinicians would argue that such tests take very little time and should be performed on every patient with neck pain. Any doubt about the integrity of the upper cervical spine ligaments should preclude the use of thrust joint manipulation. A 'safety first' attitude seems more than prudent here.

6.4.1: Alar Ligament Active Motion Test

The patient is seated and the clinician places their thumb and index or middle finger on the lamina of C2, bilaterally. The patient is asked to actively laterally flex (side-bend) to the left and right, and the clinician can gently guide this active motion with their other hand (Figure 6.4.1a). During lateral flexion of the upper cervical spine, the odontoid should remain midway between the occipital condyles because of its fixation by the alar ligaments.[42] During craniovertebral (O-C1) lateral flexion, there is combined contralateral atlantoaxial (C1-C2) rotation due to the orientation and function of the alar ligament.[43] The C2 vertebra rotates toward the side of O-C1 lateral flexion in relation to C3, which causes a relative contralateral rotation of the C1-C2 spinal segment.[44] Therefore, as the patient laterally flexes their neck to the left, the clinician should feel the spinous process of C2 moving to the right. There are no reliability statistics for this active motion test; however, the authors contend that with practice, this skill can be developed and, if lack of motion of the C2 spinous process is noted, the likelihood of a torn or damaged alar ligament should be considered. If there is a delay in the movement of the C2 spinous process into the opposite direction to lateral flexion noted, then the probability of a partial tear should be considered.

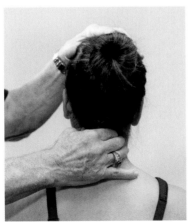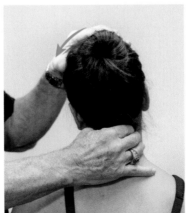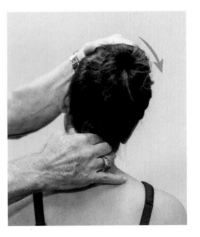

Figure 6.4.1a: Alar Ligament Active Motion Test.

6.4.2: Alar Ligament Stress Test

The passive alar ligament stress test can be performed in sitting or with the patient in supine lying (Figure 6.4.2.a). With the patient sitting, ensure the neck is in a neutral position, and that there is no side-bending of the head and neck. The clinician stabilizes the spinous process and vertebral arch of C2 with thumb and index/middle finger while placing the other hand on the patient's vertex. The clinician then attempts to passively laterally flex to the left and then right. There should be minimal to no movement in either direction, and the test should be repeated with the neck in flexion and extension to account for variation in alar ligament orientation.[45] A positive test is determined by the onset of symptoms or signs and/or an increased range of passive lateral flexion in at least two positions; neutral, flexion or extension.

Osmotherly et al[46] found there was good construct validity for the clinical tests of alar ligament integrity through the use of magnetic resonance imaging. They found that both side-bending and rotation stress testing resulted in a measurable increase in length of the contralateral alar ligament.

6.4.3: Transverse Ligament Test (Aspinall)

The transverse ligament test (also known as the anterior shear test) was first described by Wendy Aspinall in 1990,[45] and is now commonly taught in professional level physical therapist programs; however, its validity has not been established.[47] The test is performed with the patient in the supine position. The clinician supports the occiput, while the two index fingers are placed in the space between the occiput and the C2 spinous process. The head and C1 are then moved anteriorly as a unit on the cervical spine, while avoiding flexion (Figure 6.4.3a). Aspinall[45] held that no movement or symptoms should be perceived if the transverse ligament is normal, thus preventing any anterior translation of the atlas on the axis. The symptom experienced for this test to be classified as positive is a feeling the patient may have of a lump in the throat as the atlas moves toward the esophagus. The test position can be held for 10-20 seconds, while the clinician observes the patient for cardinal signs and/or swallowing difficulties.

Osmotherly et al[48] examined the anterior shear test using magnetic resonance imaging and reported a 0.41 mm mean increase in the atlantodental interval (p=0.03) with the application of the test in 16 skeletally mature healthy individuals aged 18 - 35 years.

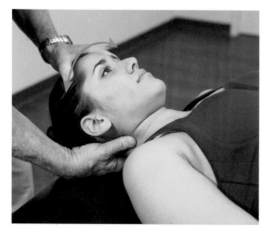

Figure 6.4.2a: Alar Ligament Stress Test.

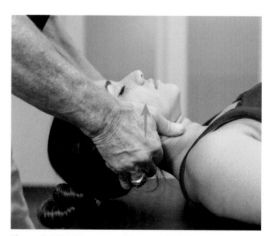

Figure 6.4.3a: Transverse Ligament Test (Aspinall).

6.4.4: Sharp-Purser test

Sharp and Purser first described a test for the clinical assessment of anterior atlantoaxial subluxation which is common in patients with rheumatoid arthritis with involvement of the cervical spine. The validity of the Sharp-Purser test in 123 patients with rheumatoid arthritis was assessed by Uitvlugt and Indenbaum.[49] They found a predictive value of 85 percent and a specificity of 96 percent, and the sensitivity was 88 percent when subluxation was greater than four mm. However, it should be remembered that these statistics apply only to a population with rheumatoid arthritis.

The original test is performed with the patient seated and the neck relaxed in a semi-flexed position. The clinician places the palm of one hand on the patient's forehead and the index finger of the other hand on the tip of the spinous process of the axis. While pressing backward with the palm, a sliding motion of the head posterior in relation to the axis is indicative of atlantoaxial instability.[49]

A modified version of the test is commonly used by clinicians in patients with neck pain, headache and/or upper extremity symptoms without rheumatoid arthritis. The modified Sharp-Purser test is one of elimination of symptoms. The test is performed in exactly the same manner; however, symptoms are assessed when the patient flexes their head to approximately 30 degrees. When a test is considered positive, patients will report symptoms (neck pain, headache, dizziness, or upper extremity paresthesia) and the symptoms are relieved with the application of the posterior sliding motion of the head relative to the axis (Figure 6.4.4a).

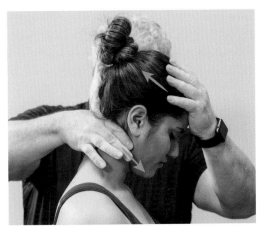

Figure 6.4.4a: Modified Sharp-Purser test.

6.4.5: Tectorial Membrane Test (Pettman's Distraction Test)

Distraction testing can be used to assess the integrity of the tectorial membrane due to its described role as a limiting factor in vertical translation.[50,51] The patient is positioned in supine with their head resting on a pillow, as this is supposed to relax the upper cervical musculature and to eliminate the stabilizing effect of the ligamentum nuchae.[47] With their lower hand, the clinician gently fixates C2 around its neural arch and cups the occiput with their upper hand (Figure 6.4.5a). A manual traction is then applied to the head, as the test is performed in three planes; neutral, flexion and extension.[45,52] It is generally accepted that some movement on application of a distraction force is normal. A positive test response is considered to be excessive vertical translation when distraction is applied, and reproduction or aggravation of the patient's symptoms (pain or paresthesia).

Osmotherly et al[48] examined the distraction test using magnetic resonance imaging and reported a 0.64 mm mean increase in the basion-dental interval ($p<0.01$) and a 1.11 mm increase in direct ligament length measurement ($p=0.02$) with the application of the test in 16 skeletally mature healthy individuals aged 18 - 35 years.

6.4.6: Lateral Shear Tests

Although it is not commonly taught in professional-level physical therapist programs, the authors find good clinical utility in the cervical lateral shear tests. The patient is placed supine with their head on a pillow. Starting from the atlantoaxial joint and working their way down, the clinician places the proximal phalanx of one index finger on the lamina above, and the proximal phalanx of the other index finger on the lamina of the segment below. Force is applied simultaneously into each lamina in attempt to produce a shear force across the spine at each segmental level (Figure 6.4.6a). The clinician should switch hands, placing the opposite hand on the superior segment and the original hand on the inferior segment at the same level. This should be repeated all the way down the cervical spine, and the clinician is looking for excessive movement along the plane of the facet and/or an empty end feel. Such finding might suggest the possibility of a hypermobility and/or instability in the cervical spine. Obviously, corroborating history will be helpful to verify this diagnosis.

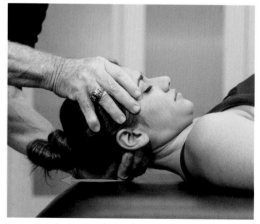

Figure 6.4.5a: Tectorial Membrane Test (Pettman's Distraction Test).

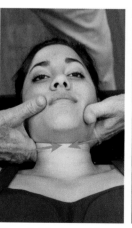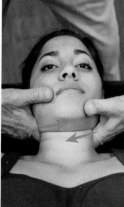

Figure 6.4.6a: Lateral Shear Tests.

6.5: Lumbar Tests

The following tests are thought to help determine the presence of lumbar segmental instability. Their clinical utility was called into question when a recent systematic review found that the majority of these tests demonstrated only limited ability to do so.[53]

6.5.1: Lumbar Anterior Shear Test

For this test, the patient is side-lying with hips flexed to about 70 degrees and knees comfortably flexed. The clinician's hands are placed over the lumbar motion segment to be tested. The patient's knees are placed into the crease of the clinician's hip, and the clinician palpates and stabilizes the targeted spinous process. Using hip contact, the clinician pushes posteriorly through the patient's knees and long the line of the femur (Figure 6.5.1a). The clinician may feel for any relative movement of the segment caudal to the segment being stabilized.

A positive test would be where the clinician feels forward motion of the cephalad segment relative to the caudal segment, and they may also note spasm in the muscles surrounding an unstable motion segment.

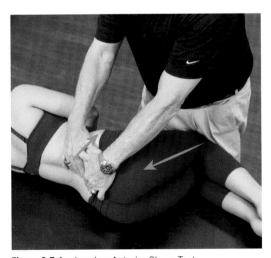

Figure 6.5.1a: Lumbar Anterior Shear Test.

6.5.2: Prone Instability Test

The prone instability test is performed with the patient prone, with the trunk supported on the examining table and the feet resting on the floor (Figure 6.5.2a). With the patient in this position, the clinician performs a posterior-to-anterior intervertebral motion test to each level of the lumbar spine. Any provocation of pain should be recorded. The patient is then asked to lift the feet slightly off the floor and the posterior-to-anterior motion is repeated. If pain was present in the resting position but subsides in the second position, the test is deemed positive.[4] The prone instability has good interrater reliability (Kappa=0.69),[54] and sensitivity and specificity reported as 0.61 and 0.57, respectively.[4]

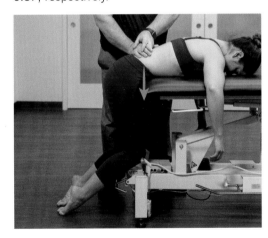

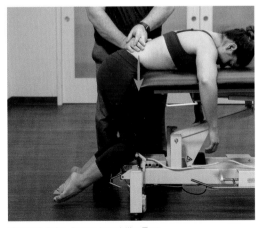

Figure 6.5.2a: Prone Instability Test.

6.5.3: Posterior Shear Test

The posterior shear test is performed with the patient standing, with hands across the lower abdomen. The clinician places one hand over the patient's crossed arms and the heel of the other hand on the patient's pelvis for stabilization. The clinician produces a posterior shear force through the patient's abdomen, and an anteriorly directed stabilizing force with the opposite hand (Figure 6.5.3a). The test can be repeated at each lumbar level by changing the point of contact of the posterior hand. A positive test occurs if familiar symptoms are provoked, and is proposed to indicate lumbar instability.[4] The posterior shear test has poor interrater reliability (Kappa=0.27),[54] and sensitivity and specificity reported as 0.57 and 0.48, respectively.[4]

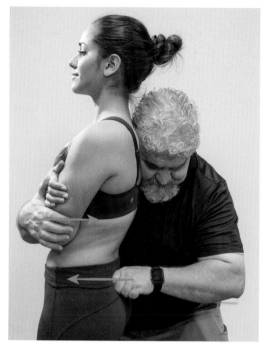

Figure 6.5.3a: Posterior Shear Test.

6.6: Key Points from Chapter 6

- Prior to delivering thrust joint manipulation to the spine, it is imperative that clinicians conduct thorough subjective (history) and objective (physical) examinations.

- Information gathered from the subjective and objective examinations should be considered in the clinical reasoning process, which might lead a clinician to consider using a thrust joint manipulation technique.

- Although the evidence suggests that many of the tests have poor intra- and interrater reliability and validity, we would urge clinicians to utilize any special tests they deem necessary and err on the side of caution prior to delivering a spinal manipulative technique (particularly in the upper cervical spine).

Chapter 6 References

1. Mitchell J, Keene D, Dyson C, Harvey L, Pruvey C, Phillips R. Is cervical spine rotation, as used in the standard vertebrobasilar insufficiency test, associated with a measureable change in intracranial vertebral artery blood flow? *Man Ther.* 2004;9(4):220-227.

2. Alshahrani A, Johnson EG, Cordett TK. Vertebral artery testing and differential diagnosis in dizzy patients. *Physical Therapy and Rehabilitation.* 2014;1(1).

3. Hunt DG, Zuberbier OA, Kozlowski AJ, et al. Reliability of the lumbar flexion, lumbar extension, and passive straight leg raise test in normal populations embedded within a complete physical examination. *Spine (Phila Pa 1976).* 2001;26(24):2714-2718.

4. Fritz JM, Piva SR, Childs JD. Accuracy of the clinical examination to predict radiographic instability of the lumbar spine. *Eur Spine J.* 2005;14(8):743-750.

5. Wainner RS, Fritz JM, Irrgang JJ, Boninger ML, Delitto A, Allison S. Reliability and diagnostic accuracy of the clinical examination and patient self-report measures for cervical radiculopathy. *Spine (Phila Pa 1976).* 2003;28(1):52-62.

6. Olson SL, O'Connor DP, Birmingham G, Broman P, Herrera L. Tender point sensitivity, range of motion, and perceived disability in subjects with neck pain. *J Orthop Sports Phys Ther.* 2000;30(1):13-20.

7. Youdas JW, Carey JR, Garrett TR. Reliability of measurements of cervical spine range of motion--comparison of three methods. *Phys Ther.* 1991;71(2):98-104; discussion 105-106.

8. Smedmark V, Wallin M, Arvidsson I. Inter-examiner reliability in assessing passive intervertebral motion of the cervical spine. Man Ther. 2000;5(2):97-101.

9. Brismée J-M, Gipson D, Ivie D, et al. Interrater Reliability of a Passive Physiological Intervertebral Motion Test in the Mid-Thoracic Spine. *Journal of Manipulative and Physiological Therapeutics.* 2006;29(5):368-373.

10. Keating JC, Jr., Bergmann TF, Jacobs GE, Finer BA, Larson K. Interexaminer reliability of eight evaluative dimensions of lumbar segmental abnormality. *J Manipulative Physiol Ther.* 1990;13(8):463-470.

11. Matyas TA, Bach TM. The Reliability of Selected Techniques in Clinical Arthrometrics. *Australian Journal of Physiotherapy.* 1985;31(5):175-199.

12. Phillips DR, Twomey LT. A comparison of manual diagnosis with a diagnosis established by a uni-level lumbar spinal block procedure. *Manual Therapy.* 1996;1(2):82-87.

13. Piva SR, Erhard RE, Childs JD, Browder DA. Inter-tester reliability of passive intervertebral and active movements of the cervical spine. *Manual Therapy.* 2006;11(4):321-330.

14. van Trijffel E, Oostendorp RAB, Lindeboom R, Bossuyt PMM, Lucas C. Perceptions and use of passive intervertebral motion assessment of the spine: A survey among physiotherapists specializing in manual therapy. *Manual Therapy.* 2009;14(3):243-251.

15. Banks K. Geoffrey D. Maitland, 1924–2010. *Physical Therapy.* 2010;90(3):326-326.

16. Johnston WL, Allan BR, Hendra JL, et al. Interexaminer study of palpation in detecting location of spinal segmental dysfunction. *J Am Osteopath Assoc.* 1983;82(11):839-845.

17. Cooperstein R. Interexaminer reliability of the Johnston and Friedman percussion scan of the thoracic spine: secondary data analysis using modified methods. *J Chiropr Med.* 2012;11(3):154-159.

18. Ghoukassian M, Nicholls B, McLaughlin P. Inter-examiner reliability of the Johnson and Friedman percussion scan of the thoracic spine. *Journal of Osteopathic Medicine.* 2001;4(1):15-20.

19. Fryer G, Morris T, Gibbons P. The relationship between palpation of thoracic tissues and deep paraspinal muscle thickness. *International Journal of Osteopathic Medicine.*8(1):22-28.

20. Hartman L. *Thoracic tap test.* Personal Communication; 2015.

21. Laslett M. The value of the physical examination in diagnosis of painful sacroiliac joint pathologies. *Spine (Phila Pa 1976).* 1998;23(8):962-964.

22. Laslett M. Pain provocation tests for diagnosis of sacroiliac joint pain. *Aust J Physiother.* 2006;52(3):229.

23. Laslett M. Evidence-based diagnosis and treatment of the painful sacroiliac joint. *J Man Manip Ther.* 2008;16(3):142-152.

24. Laslett M, Williams M. The reliability of selected pain provocation tests for sacroiliac joint pathology. *Spine (Phila Pa 1976).* 1994;19(11):1243-1249.

25. Laslett M, Aprill CN, McDonald B, Young SB. Diagnosis of sacroiliac joint pain: validity of individual provocation tests and composites of tests. *Man Ther.* 2005;10(3):207-218.

26. Laslett M, Aprill CN, McDonald B. Provocation sacroiliac joint tests have validity in the diagnosis of sacroiliac joint pain. *Arch Phys Med Rehabil.* 2006;87(6):874; author reply 874-875.

27. Hancock MJ, Maher CG, Latimer J, et al. Systematic review of tests to identify the disc, SIJ or facet joint as the source of low back pain. *Eur Spine J.* 2007;16(10):1539-1550.

28. Arnbak B, Jurik AG, Jensen RK, Schiottz-Christensen B, van der Wurff P, Jensen TS. The diagnostic value of three sacroiliac joint pain provocation tests for sacroiliitis identified by magnetic resonance imaging. *Scand J Rheumatol.* 2016:1-8.

29. Szadek KM, van der Wurff P, van Tulder MW, Zuurmond WW, Perez RS. Diagnostic validity of criteria for sacroiliac joint pain: a systematic review. *J Pain.* 2009;10(4):354-368.

30. van der Wurff P. Clinical diagnostic tests for the sacroiliac joint: motion and palpation tests. *Aust J Physiother.* 2006;52(4):308.

31. van der Wurff P, Buijs EJ, Groen GJ. A multitest regimen of pain provocation tests as an aid to reduce unnecessary minimally invasive sacroiliac joint procedures. *Arch Phys Med Rehabil.* 2006;87(1):10-14.

32. Kokmeyer DJ, Van der Wurff P, Aufdemkampe G, Fickenscher TC. The reliability of multitest regimens with sacroiliac pain provocation tests. *J Manipulative Physiol Ther.* 2002;25(1):42-48.

33. van der Wurff P, Meyne W, Hagmeijer RH. Clinical tests of the sacroiliac joint. *Man Ther.* 2000;5(2):89-96.

34. van der Wurff P, Hagmeijer RH, Meyne W. Clinical tests of the sacroiliac joint. A systematic methodological review. Part 1: Reliability. *Man Ther.* 2000;5(1):30-36.

35. Fortin JD, Dwyer AP, West S, Pier J. Sacroiliac joint: pain referral maps upon applying a new injection/arthrography technique. Part I: Asymptomatic volunteers. *Spine (Phila Pa 1976).* 1994;19(13):1475-1482.

36. Fortin JD, Falco FJ. The Fortin finger test: an indicator of sacroiliac pain. *Am J Orthop (Belle Mead NJ).* 1997;26(7):477-480.

37. Murakami E, Aizawa T, Noguchi K, Kanno H, Okuno H, Uozumi H. Diagram specific to sacroiliac joint pain site indicated by one-finger test. *J Orthop Sci.* 2008;13(6):492-497.

38. Gaenslen FJ. Sacro-iliac arthrodesis: Indications, author's technic and end-results. *Journal of the American Medical Association.* 1927;89(24):2031-2035.

39. Cook C, Brismee JM, Fleming R, Sizer PS, Jr. Identifiers suggestive of clinical cervical spine instability: a Delphi study of physical therapists. *Phys Ther.* 2005;85(9):895-906.

40. Cattrysse E, Swinkels RA, Oostendorp RA, Duquet W. Upper cervical instability: are clinical tests reliable? *Man Ther.* 1997;2(2):91-97.

41. Olson KA, Paris SV, Spohr C, Gorniak G. Radiographic Assessment and Reliability Study of the Craniovertebral Sidebending Test. *Journal of Manual & Manipulative Therapy.* 1998;6(2):87-96.

42. Penning L. Normal movements of the cervical spine. *AJR Am J Roentgenol.* 1978;130(2):317-326.

43. Mimura M, Moriya H, Watanabe T, Takahashi K, Yamagata M, Tamaki T. Three-dimensional motion analysis of the cervical spine with special reference to the axial rotation. *Spine (Phila Pa 1976).* 1989;14(11):1135-1139.

44. Ishii T, Mukai Y, Hosono N, et al. Kinematics of the subaxial cervical spine in rotation in vivo three-dimensional analysis. *Spine (Phila Pa 1976).* 2004;29(24):2826-2831.

45. Aspinall W. Clinical testing for the craniovertebral hypermobility syndrome. *J Orthop Sports Phys Ther.* 1990;12(2):47-54.

46. Osmotherly PG, Rivett DA, Rowe LJ. Construct validity of clinical tests for alar ligament integrity: an evaluation using magnetic resonance imaging. *Phys Ther.* 2012;92(5):718-725.

47. Pettman E. Stress tests of the craniovertebral joints. In: Boyling J, Palastanga N, eds. *Grieve's Modern Manual Therapy: The Vertebral Column.* Edinburgh, UK: Churchill Livingstone; 1994:529-538.

48. Osmotherly PG, Rivett DA, Rowe LJ. The anterior shear and distraction tests for craniocervical instability. An evaluation using magnetic resonance imaging. *Manual Therapy.* 2012;17(5):416-421.

49. Uitvlugt G, Indenbaum S. Clinical assessment of atlantoaxial instability using the Sharp-Purser test. *Arthritis Rheum.* 1988;31(7):918-922.

50. Werne S. Factors limiting the range of movement of the craniovertebral joints. *Acta Orthopaedica Scandinavia Suppl.* 1957;23(1):38-62.

51. White AA, Panjabi MM. *Clinical Biomechanics of the Spine.* 2nd Ed. ed. Philadelphia, PA: J.B. Lippincott Company; 1990.

52. Hing W, Reid D. Cervical spine management. Pre-screening requirement for New Zealand. *New Zealand Manipulative Physiotherapists Association.* 2004.

53. Alqarni AM, Schneiders AG, Hendrick PA. Clinical tests to diagnose lumbar segmental instability: a systematic review. *J Orthop Sports Phys Ther.* 2011;41(3):130-140.

54. Hicks GE, Fritz JM, Delitto A, Mishock J. Interrater reliability of clinical examination measures for identification of lumbar segmental instability. *Arch Phys Med Rehabil.* 2003;84(12):1858-1864.

Chapter 7

Thrust Joint Manipulation Techniques for the Spine

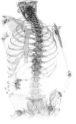

7.1: Chapter Objectives

In this chapter, we provide step-by-step instructions for the performance of thrust joint manipulation techniques we have regularly used in the treatment of dysfunction in the spine. Of course, there are many other techniques that we could include, but as stated earlier, it is not the goal of this textbook to present every thrust joint technique that can be performed on the spine. Instead, we are describing those techniques with which we have personally had the greatest clinical success.

For each technique, we provide clear instructions for patient position, therapist position, contact points, position for the thrust, and application of the thrust. There are also photos and videos of each technique to provide visual aids to learning (see instructions below for access to videos). Finally, we provide some notes on fine tuning and keys to successfully achieving joint cavitation with each technique.

Terminology:
The particular name that we, as clinicians, might give to specific manipulative techniques varies greatly depending upon where we practice and where we learned the techniques. The terminology we use tends to be understandable only to those of us who

have undergone the same specific training. Indeed, it has been said that manipulation is often obscured by illusive and ill-defined terminology.[1] In an attempt to rectify this problem, in February 2007, the American Academy of Orthopaedic Manual Physical Therapists (AAOMPT) formed a task force to standardize manual therapy terminology, starting with the intervention of manipulation. That task force, headed by Dr. Paul Mintken and colleagues, proposed a nomenclature intended to standardize and clarify the terminology used in describing specific manipulative techniques.[2] They recommended the use of six key characteristics:[2]

1. Rate of force application

2. Location in the range of available movement

3. Direction of force

4. Target of the force

5. Relative structural movement

6. Patient position

Using these six key characteristics, the lumbar rotation manipulation performed in side-lying with the spine in neutral or slight extension (commonly known as the 'lumbar roll'), becomes a "high-velocity, end-range, right-rotational force to the lower lumbar spine on the upper lumbar spine in a right side-lying, left lower thoracic lumbar side-bent position."[2] So, how popular has this recommended terminology become? How widespread is its use? We would argue that this recommended terminology has not been widely adopted, and suggest that it may well be because of the lengthy descriptions required.

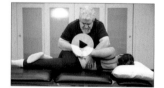

Video techniques found in Chapter 7 can be accessed at this web page:

OPTP.com/tjm-videos
Username: tjm
Password: techniques

Effective teaching of manual skills:

The effectiveness of different teaching and learning approaches in skills laboratories is still debated in the literature.[3] In the past, teaching technical skills such as thrust joint manipulation has been based upon the paradigm of learning by doing, which is commonly known as the 'See one, do one' approach.[4] Such an approach makes the assumption that trainees can become proficient and independent in the performance of a specific technique after observing its performance once by an expert clinician or teacher.[5,6] However, there is documented criticism of the 'See one, do one' approach as inadequate in maintaining required patient safety standards because of the lack of supervision, reflection on action, performance evaluation and structured feedback.[7,8] This led to the development of a five-step model of teaching clinical skills,[9] which was later refined as Peyton's four-step approach.[10] The approach consists of four teaching steps: demonstration; deconstruction; comprehension; and performance. It has been documented as effective in laboratories for teaching procedural skills,[11] and was recently shown to be superior to the 'See one, do one' approach in physiotherapy students learning to perform C1-C2 passive mobilization.[12]

Based on this evidence, we have created video presentations of the thrust joint manipulation skills that will follow Peyton's four-step approach to teaching a clinical skill. Essentially it involves:

1. Teacher demonstrating the skill at normal speed, with no words (Demonstration)

2. Teacher demonstrating the skill while describing the steps (Deconstruction)

3. Teacher demonstrating the skill while the learner describes the steps (Comprehension)

4. Learner performing the skill while describing the steps (Performance)

The videos that will accompany this book will only show the first two steps. We will first perform each thrust joint manipulation technique at normal speed without any words to show what we are doing (Step 1), and then we will repeat the technique more slowly. This second time, we will describe each of the steps (Step 2), and then, we recommend that you replay the video with the sound muted so that you, the learner, can describe the steps (Step 3). We would then encourage you to move to Step 4, performance of the technique, at your earliest convenience.

7.2.1: Minimal Leverage Gap Thrust to the OA Joint

Description: This technique is performed with the patient in supine and where the therapist contacts the posterior arch of the atlas (C1) with their second metacarpophalangeal (MCP) joint. Slack is taken up through the tissues with the applicator hand. The opposite hand takes up a chin hold. The thrust is directed through the posterior arch of the atlas toward the opposite eye while the opposite forearm provides counterforce to the side of the head. The result will be a gapping of C1 on the occiput on the same side.

When to use: To restore motion of the OA joint on the ipsilateral side using a translation motion to gap the joint. This is most useful when you want to avoid torsion and the joint fixation is not too severe.

Primary muscles activated: Shoulder adductors and protractors with the thrusting arm. Shoulder adductors of non-thrusting arm.

Suggested tests prior to thrust:
- Alar ligament tests.
- Transverse ligament tests.
- Pre-manipulative hold.
- Sharp-Purser (if indicated).
- Tectorial membrane test (as needed).
- PPIVMs/PAIVMs.

Patient position (Figure 7.2.1a):
- Supine with head on a pillow.

Therapist position (Figure 7.2.1a):
- Standing at the corner of table on the side to be treated (in this case, the right).

Contact points:
- Second MCP of your right hand contacts posterior arch of C1 on the right side.
- The head is cradled with the left hand using a gentle chin hold.

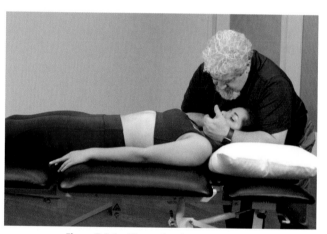

Figure 7.2.1a: The patient is supine with head on a pillow and the therapist stands at the corner of the table on the side to be treated and takes up a chin hold.

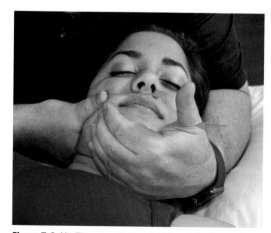

Figure 7.2.1b: Thrust, with the right hand, is directed toward the left eye while the left forearm applies a counterforce in the opposite direction.

Position for thrust:

- Position the patient diagonally with their head and neck toward you, to get them as close to you as possible.

- Rotate the head just enough to allow access to the posterior arch with your thrusting hand.

- Introduce a small amount of side-bending to the right and minimal rotation to the left.

Application of the thrust (Figure 7.2.1b)**:**

- Once you have gathered the forces by sequentially adding levers, provide a few mini-thrusts to test the barrier.

- This can be a difficult technique as it is not easy to feel the accumulation of the barrier.

- The thrust, with the right hand, is directly toward the left eye while your left forearm applies a counterforce in the opposite direction.

Fine-tuning and keys for success:

- It is helpful to have the patient lay diagonally so that you lessen the distance you have to reach to apply the thrust.

- Have the patient move their feet to the corner of the table while having the head at the corner of the table closest to you.

- Avoid having the patient side-bend their trunk as this can change the dynamics of what you are trying to do and can be uncomfortable for them.

- Standing as close to the patient as you can allows you to put compression or traction through the patient's head, if needed.

- The table height should be set so that it is about waist high.

- Make sure you use the correct contact points (posterior arch of C1 with your second MCP).

- With the chin hold technique, you need to tuck the corner of the patient's head in that space between the anterior deltoid and the lateral pectoral muscle of the non-thrusting side.

- Because this is an upper cervical technique, minimal levers will be needed to get a proper purchase on the atlas and avoid injury to the patient.

- Compression with the opposite forearm against the patient's head will help minimize any unwanted motion and will also serve to apply an adequate counterforce to ensure greater success.

- It is critical that you do not lock the joint. This technique is based on speed and most of all, direction.

- You will have a hard time feeling the accumulation of the barrier with this technique. Hence, another reason speed is critical.

- Do not lift the patient's head off the pillow. In the authors' experience, patients are less tense when they are resting on the pillow than when they are held in the air.

Description: This supine cradle hold technique moves the occiput relative to C1 using a scooping motion along the plane of the joint. The occiput is contacted by the proximal phalanx of the index finger. The other hand cradles the head. The occiput is thrusted in a scooping motion of the occiput on C1 along the plane of the joint toward the opposite eye. This technique is commonly used to restore upper cervical extension. However, Gibbons and Tehan use this technique to restore motion regardless of whether the OA is fixed in flexion or extension.

When to use: Primarily used to restore unilateral extension of the occiput on the atlas. Can be used to restore general movement at the OA joint.

Primary muscles activated: Shoulder adductors and protractors with the thrusting arm. Shoulder extensors and retractors of non-thrusting arm.

Suggested tests prior to thrust:
- Alar ligament tests.
- Transverse ligament tests.
- Pre-manipulative hold.
- Sharp-Purser (if indicated).
- Tectorial membrane test (as needed).
- PPIVMs/PAIVMs.

Patient position (Figure 7.2.2a)**:**
- Supine with head on a pillow.

Therapist position (Figure 7.2.2a)**:**
- Standing at head of table toward the side you will treat (in this case, the right side).

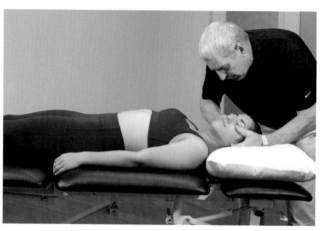

Figure 7.2.2a: Patient supine with head on a pillow and therapist standing at head of table toward the side to be treated (right side).

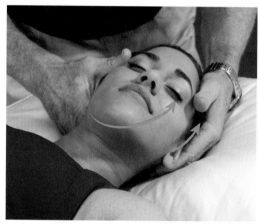

Figure 7.2.2b: Thrust is applied in a scooping arc along the plane of the OA joint toward the opposite (left) eye. The left hand assists with the motion in the same direction.

Contact points:
- Proximal phalanx of index finger contacts the base of the occiput posterior and medial to the mastoid on the affected side.

- The head is cradled with the opposite hand.

Position for thrust:
- Move the patient diagonally toward you to get them as close to you as possible.

- Introduce a primary lever of left rotation enough to where you are able to position the thrusting hand on the right occiput.

- Add right side-bending and a little extension. The latter two are really minimal.

Application of the thrust (Figure 7.2.2b)**:**
- Once you have gathered the forces by sequentially adding levers, provide a few mini-thrusts to test the barrier.

- Fine-tune and improve focusing at the barrier by adding compressions and/or traction as needed.

- The thrust is applied in a scooping arc toward the opposite (left) eye.

Fine-tuning and keys for success:
- It is helpful to have patient lay diagonally so that you lessen the distance you have to reach to apply the thrust.

- Have the patient move their feet to the corner of the table while having the head at the corner of the table closest to you.

- Avoid having the patient side-bend their trunk as it can change the dynamics of what you are trying to do and can be uncomfortable for them.

- Standing as close to the patient as you can allows you to put compression or traction through the patient's head.

- The table height should be set so that it is about waist high.

- Make sure you use the correct contact points (lower occiput with the proximal phalanx of the index finger).

- This is a two-handed technique. If you use a chin hold technique, you need to tuck the corner of the patient's head in that space between the anterior deltoid and the lateral pectoral muscle of the non-thrusting side.

- Rotation will vary from patient to patient depending on their flexibility. Never introduce excessive rotation. 45 degrees is probably adequate.

- Be careful not to add too much motion to the remaining components. Because there is very little motion required to engage the barrier there, one might cause either injury or discomfort to the patient if the subsequent levers are excessive.

- Adding additional components such as traction or compression through the skull may help to further focus your forces and guarantee greater success.

- It is critical that you do not lock the joint. This technique is based on speed and most of all, direction.

- Do not lift the patient's head off the pillow. In the authors' experience patients are less tense when they are resting on the pillow than when they are held in air.

7.2.3: Scoop Technique to Move C1 Anteriorly on Occiput (OA Flexion)

Description: This supine chin hold technique moves the C1 relative to the occiput using a scooping motion along the plane of the joint. In our experience, most people are stuck in extension in the upper C spine. This thrust is directed with therapist's proximal phalanx of the index finger contacting the posterior arch of C1 and moves it toward the patient's opposite eye. The opposite hand cradles the head and aids in the scooping motion.

When to use: Primarily used to restore unilateral flexion of the occiput on the atlas. Can be used to restore general movement at the OA joint.

Primary muscles activated: Shoulder adductors and protractors with the thrusting arm. Shoulder extensors and retractors of non-thrusting arm.

Suggested tests prior to thrust:
- Alar ligament tests.
- Transverse ligament tests.
- Pre-manipulative hold.
- Sharp-Purser (if indicated).
- Tectorial membrane test (as needed).
- PPIVMs/PAIVMs.

Patient position (Figure 7.2.3a):
- Supine with head on a pillow.

Therapist position (Figure 7.2.3a):
- Standing at head of table toward the side you will treat (in this case, the right side).

Contact points:
- Proximal phalanx of index finger contacts the posterior arch of C1 on the affected side.

- The head is cradled with the opposite hand using a chin hold.

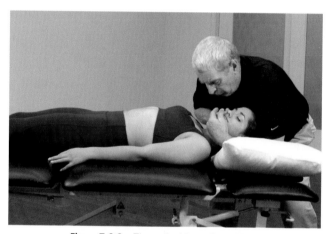

Figure 7.2.3a: The patient is supine with head on a pillow and the therapist stands at the corner of the table on the side to be treated and takes up a chin hold.

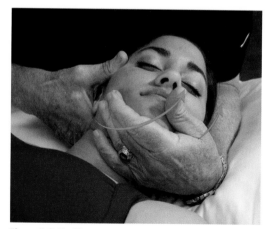

Figure 7.2.3b: Thrust, using both hands, is applied in a scooping arc along the plane of the joint toward the patient's opposite (left) eye. The left hand and forearm assist with the motion in the same direction.

Position for thrust:
- Move the patient diagonally toward you to get them as close to you as possible.

- Introduce a primary lever of left rotation enough to where you are able to position the thrusting hand on the posterior arch of C1.

- Add right side-bending and a little extension. The latter two are really minimal.

Application of the thrust (Figure 7.2.3b)**:**
- Once you have gathered the forces by sequentially adding levers, provide a few mini-thrusts to test the barrier.

- Fine-tune and improve focusing at the barrier by adding compressions and/or traction as needed.

- The thrust is applied in a scooping arc toward the opposite (left) eye.

Fine-tuning and keys for success:
- It is helpful to have patient lay diagonally so that you lessen the distance you have to reach to apply the thrust.

- Have the patient move their feet to the corner of the table while having the head at the corner of the table closest to you.

- Avoid having the patient side-bend their trunk as it can change the dynamics of what you are trying to do and can be uncomfortable for them.

- Standing as close to the patient as you can allows you to put compression or traction through the patient's head.

- The table height should be set so that it is about waist high.

- Make sure you use the correct contact points (posterior arch of C1 with the proximal phalanx of the index finger).

- This is a two-handed technique. With the chin hold technique, you need to tuck the corner of the patient's head in that space between the anterior deltoid and the lateral pectoral muscle of the non-thrusting side.

- Rotation will vary from patient to patient depending on their flexibility. Never introduce excessive rotation. 45 degrees is probably adequate.

- Be careful not to add too much motion to the remaining components. Because there is very little motion required to engage the barrier there, one might cause either injury or discomfort to the patient if the subsequent levers are excessive.

- Adding additional components such as traction or compression through the skull may help to further focus your forces and guarantee greater success.

- It is critical that you do not lock the joint. This technique is based on speed and most of all, direction.

- Do not lift the patient's head off the pillow. In the authors' experience patients are less tense when they are resting on the pillow than when they are held in air.

Description: This is one of the gentler techniques with the patient in a supine position on the table. The thrusting hand makes contact on the occiput. Small amounts of ipsilateral side-bending, contralateral rotation and extension are introduced to allow the thrusting hand to get a good purchase on the occiput. The thrusting arm rests on the patient's lateral chest anterior to the shoulder. A small impulse is made toward the vertex of the skull. The opposite forearm compressing the patient's skull into your chest aids in the thrust.

Primary muscles activated: Shoulder adductors of thrusting side. Shoulder abductors of opposite extremity.

When to use: To restore motion to the OA joint that is fixed. Should not be used if you suspect an instability or hypermobility below the level to be treated.

Suggested tests prior to thrust:
- Alar ligament tests.
- Transverse ligament tests.
- Pre-manipulative hold.
- Sharp-Purser (if indicated).
- Tectorial membrane test (as needed).
- PPIVMs/PAIVMs.

Patient position (Figure 7.2.4a):
- Supine on table with head resting on pillow.

Therapist position (Figure 7.2.4a):
- Standing to the side of the table near the patient's head and shoulders.

- Therapist faces toward the head of the table.

- The leg on the side of the primary thrusting hand is back.

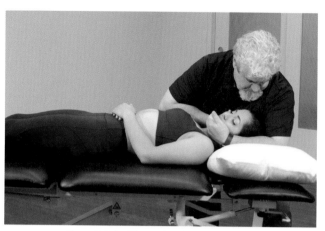

Figure 7.2.4a: The patient is supine with head on a pillow and the therapist stands to the side of the table near the patient's head and shoulder. The thrusting arm rests on the patient's lateral chest anterior to the shoulder.

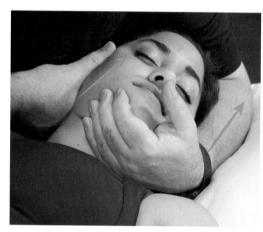

Figure 7.2.4b: A very small amplitude thrust is applied into the occiput toward the vertex of the patient's skull.

Contact points:

- Therapist contacts the underside of the ipsilateral occiput with the second MCP joint.

- The opposite hand and arm assumes a light chin hold.

Position for thrust:

- Introduce a small amount of ipsilateral side-bending at the occiput on C1.

- This is followed by the introduction of a small amount of contralateral rotation and extension.

Application of the thrust (Figure 7.2.4b)**:**

- A very small amplitude thrust is applied into the occiput toward the vertex of the patient's skull.

Fine tuning and keys to success:

- Patient should be as close to the edge of the table as possible so as to allow easy access to the segment by the therapist.

- Table height should be set so the therapist can bend easily at the waist without being placed in a biomechanical disadvantage to perform the technique.

- This is a chin hold technique. Minimal pressure is placed around the chin so as to avoid potential irritation of the TMJ.

- Having the non-thrusting forearm compress the patient's head into your chest compensates for this.

- The best way to take up the slack is to gently move toward the patient's vertex. You will know when you have reached the barrier when the nose nods forward.

- It is critical that this thrust is quick but with a very low amplitude.

- The force should not move the patient's body much but just cause a nodding at the nose.

- This technique can also be performed with the patient in side-lying (Figures 7.2.4c and 7.2.4d).

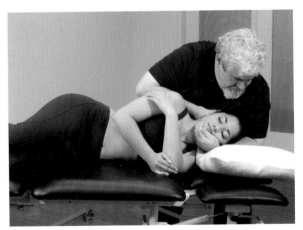

Figure 7.2.4c: In the side-lying position, the thrusting arm is behind the patient's shoulder.

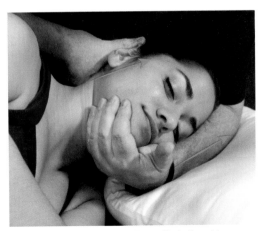

Figure 7.2.4d: The same small amplitude thrust is applied into the occiput toward the vertex of the patient's skull.

7.2.5: Atlanto-Axial (AA) Rotation Thrust – Cradle Hold

Description: The patient is supine with their head on a pillow. The therapist grasps the patient gently, applying the proximal phalanx of the second finger to the lamina behind the transverse process of C1. The opposite hand is wrapped around the chin and the patient's head is tucked between the therapist's lateral pectoral and anterior deltoid area. Contralateral rotation is introduced followed by secondary levers of ipsilateral side-bending and slight extension prior to the thrust. Other levers are added as needed to engage the barrier further. This is a two-handed technique in which the non-thrusting hand is critical for speed and control. The thrusting hand moves the patient into the primary lever of rotation while the opposite hand and forearm assist with rotation by moving into the pillow simultaneously. The chin hold is an option for performing this technique.

Primary muscles activated: Elbow flexors, shoulder adductors and elevators on the thrusting side. Forearm supinators, shoulder adductors and depressors of the non-thrusting arm.

When to use: To restore rotation at the AA joint that is fixed. Should not be used if you suspect an instability or hypermobility at the level to be treated.

Suggested tests prior to thrust:
- Sharp-Purser
- Alar ligament tests
- Transverse ligament tests
- Tectorial membrane test (as needed)
- Pre-manipulative hold
- PPIVMs/PAIVMs

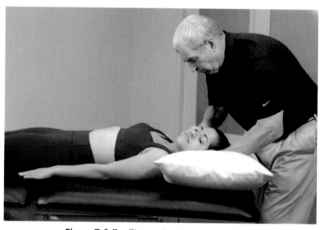

Figure 7.2.5a: The patient is supine with head on a pillow and the therapist stands to the side of the patient's head or at a 45-degree angle to the patient's head on the thrusting side.

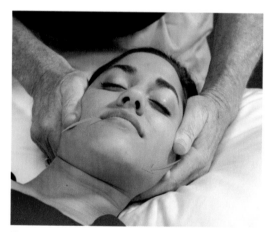

Figure 7.2.5b: Using both hands, the thrust is applied toward the patient's mouth.

Patient position (Figure 7.2.5a):
- Supine on table with head resting on pillow.

Therapist position (Figure 7.2.5a):
- Standing either to the side of the patient's head or at a 45-degree angle to the patient's head on the thrusting side

- The leg on the side of the primary thrusting hand is back.

Contact points:
- Therapist contacts the posterior lamina of C1 with the proximal phalanx of the second finger.

- The opposite hand and arm assumes a light cradle hold.

- An alternative contact can be the chin hold with the opposite hand.

- Primary lever of contralateral rotation is introduced until you feel the lamina of the superior segment come into your proximal phalanx of the thrusting hand.

- Ipsilateral side-bending to the level is then followed by adding slight extension.

- Translation, traction, additional compressions vertically and horizontally may be added to engage the barrier further.

Position for the thrust:
- Primary lever of contralateral rotation is introduced until you feel the lamina of C1 come into the proximal phalanx of the thrusting hand.

- Ipsilateral side-bending to the level is introduced followed by adding slight extension.

- Translation, traction, additional compressions vertically and horizontally may be added to engage the barrier further.

Application of thrust (Figure 7.2.5b):
- After gathering all the forces with both hands, the primary thrust is into rotation.

- Direction of the thrust is towards the patient's mouth

Fine-tuning and keys to success:
- Contact is made with your non-thrusting forearm primarily. Compressing the patient's head into your chest allows better control.

- The hand on the chin is only resting around the chin and should not be used to apply additional force or leverage.

- It is important not to lock down to the joint but to accumulate tension at C1

- Compression of the patient's head into your chest is critical prior to initiating this technique. The thrust is not initiated through the chin but with the thrusting hand and opposite forearm.

- The opposite (non-thrusting) forearm must participate for this technique to be successful.

- Less rotation and sidebending is needed because C1's more superior location requires less of either

- A helpful hint: Just after introduction of all the additional components and just prior to applying the thrust, abduct the index finger into C1.

7.2.6: Seated OA Thrust Technique (Rotation)

Description: This technique is favored by both authors to move the OA joint. It is considered one of the safer techniques to move the upper cervical spine because of the minimal amount of motion required to restore motion. It places very little or no stress on the cervical vascular structures. It is a minimal lever technique. The patient is seated. The therapist contacts the patient's head with the forearm and the anterior portion of the transverse process of C1 with the middle finger. Compression with the forearm moves the patient into ipsilateral side-bending and a little contralateral rotation to the affected/treated side. It is most effective to bend from the top down to engage the side-bending barrier. The body should be used to circumduct the patient's head and neck to further engage the barrier. Adding slight extension or flexion followed by some traction should allow for adequate engagement of the barrier. After engaging the barrier by adding components, the thrust is accomplished by rapid abduction of both arms.

When to use: To restore motion unilaterally at the occiput on C1.

Primary muscle activated: Shoulder abductors bilaterally. Shoulder extensors used to compress patient's head into the therapist's chest.

Suggested tests prior to thrust:
- Alar ligament tests.
- Transverse ligament tests.
- Pre-manipulative hold.
- Sharp-Purser (if indicated).
- Tectorial membrane test (as needed).
- PPIVMs/PAIVMs.

Patient position (Figure 7.2.6a):
- Seated on low stool, chair or table.

Therapist position (Figure 7.2.6a):
- Standing behind the patient's contralateral shoulder and making contact with the scapula.

Contact points:
- Lateral cranium just above the zygoma with medial forearm.

- Anterior to the C1 transverse process with the middle finger of the lower hand.

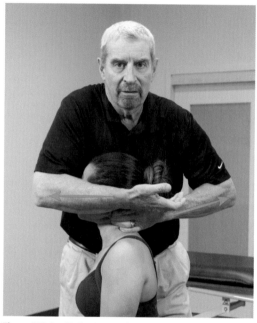

Figure 7.2.6a: Patient seated on a low chair and therapist stands behind the patient's contralateral shoulder (in this case right shoulder).

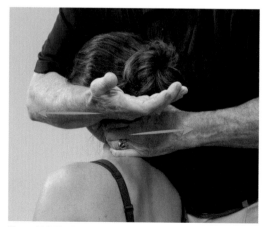

Figure 7.2.6b: Thrust is accomplished by simultaneously abducting both arms while maintaining both contact points.

Position for the thrust:
- Pull patient toward you. Compression with forearm is essential against the side of the skull into your chest.

- The fully-supinated forearm compresses the head into the therapist's chest, automatically introducing ipsilateral side-bending with contralateral rotation relative to the side being targeted.

- Add further ipsilateral side-bending by bending from the top down using your body.

- Additional levers of extension or flexion are added with traction to further engage the barrier.

Application of the thrust (Figure 7.2.6b):
- Final engagement of the barrier is done by circumduction of the patient at the level using your body against the patient's.

- The thrust is accomplished by simultaneously abducting both arms while engaging both contact points.

- The middle finger applies pressure at the instant of the thrust application.

Fine-tuning and keys to success:
- The patient should be seated at a level so that the top of their head comes no higher than the mid-chest of the therapist so as to place the patient in the optimal position of applying the technique.

- Make sure the patient is seated with no back support for easier access. If they are in a chair, have the patient sit sideways so they are not resting on the chair back.

- Therapist needs to stand as close as possible so as to be able to move patient when you move your body. This will help when you are applying circumduction.

- It is important that the arm is fully supinated and is applying compression of the head into the therapist's chest. This helps prevent the tendency to reach around the patient's skull for more leverage.

- DO NOT grab patient behind the occiput as you risk injury to the patient by increasing the lever arm around the skull.

- Use only light touch when initially contacting the anterior transverse process of C1 as this is very tender.

- The C1 transverse process is only engaged at the instant the thrust is performed.

- It is recommended that you bend from the top down to engage the barrier. Some of this barrier in side-bending will already be taken up naturally with compression of the patient's head into your chest.

- Speed is critical here. You are rapidly contracting the abductors of both shoulders.

- Adding traction after circumduction as the final component seems to guarantee the greatest success.

- Using your body to move the patient helps you feel the barriers more successfully.

- It may be helpful to perform a few mini thrusts prior to application of the actual thrust.

7.3: Middle Cervical Spine

7.3.1: Mid-cervical Spine Upslope – Cradle Hold

Description: This is a technique that uses rotation as the primary lever. It is a two-handed technique in which the non-thrusting hand is critical for speed and control. The patient is supine with their head on a pillow. The therapist applies the proximal phalanx of their index finger onto the lamina behind the transverse process of the affected segment. A primary lever of contralateral rotation is introduced, followed by ipsilateral side-bending and slight extension. Other levers such as translation, longitudinal compression and traction, etc. may be added. The non-thrusting hand is placed on the other side of the head. A thrust into a small amount of rotation is applied once the barrier is fully engaged with the addition of the other levers. The thrusting hand moves the patient into the primary lever of rotation while the opposite hand assists with rotation by moving into the pillow simultaneously.

When to use: Pain with rotation and/or side-bending to the same side, or loss of unilateral rotation and side-bending to the same side.

Primary muscles activated: Elbow flexors, forearm pronators, and shoulder protractors of thrusting arm. Forearm supinators and to a lesser degree, elbow extensors.

Suggested tests prior to thrust:
- AROM.
- Quadrant tests.
- Compression/traction tests.
- PAIVMs/PPIVMs.
- Shear tests.
- Pre-manipulative hold.

Patient position (Figure 7.3.1a):
- Supine with head on a pillow.

Therapist position (Figure 7.3.1a):
- Standing at head of table on the thrusting side.

Contacts points:
- Proximal phalanx of second finger contacts lamina behind transverse process of the superior segment.

- The opposite hand moves to the side of the head. The therapist's web space should be just behind the patient's ear.

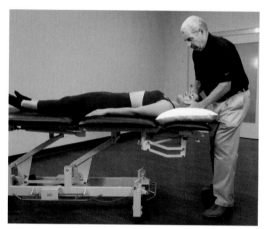

Figure 7.3.1a: Patient supine with head on a pillow and therapist standing at head of table on the side to be thrusted.

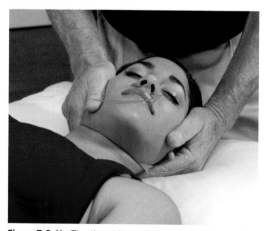

Figure 7.3.1b: The thrust is applied along the plane of the facet joint and into rotation using both hands.

Position for the thrust:
- Primary lever of contralateral rotation is introduced until you feel the lamina of the superior segment come into your proximal phalanx of the thrusting hand.

- Ipsilateral side-bending to the level is then followed by adding slight extension.

- Translation, traction, additional compressions, vertically and horizontally, may be added to engage the barrier further.

Application of the thrust (Figure 7.3.1b)**:**
- The thrust is applied along the plane of the facet joint and into rotation.

- The opposite hand drops or is thrown into the pillow at the same time.

Fine-tuning and keys to success:
- It is important to have the patient's head resting on a pillow to minimize tension in the neck that often occurs when lifting the head or having the head completely off the table.

- Have the patient get as close to the top of the table as possible. This allows the therapist to add vertical compression with their trunk.

- The table should be at a level where the therapist can handle the patient's head without much bend in their elbows when they are standing erect.

- Make sure your contact on the segment to be moved is back on the lamina of the superior segment.

- Keep the non-thrusting hand up along the side of the skull above the ear for better control with this technique.

- It is important not to lock down to the joint but to accumulate tension at the desired level.

- It is our experience that if you are getting too much activation of the sternocleidomastoid muscle on the thrust side, then you have introduced too much rotation as your primary lever.

- A good way to start rotation is to allow the head to fall into rotation onto the non-thrusting hand.

- Because this is an upslope technique, it is critical that this is a rotation around the vertex of the head toward the opposite eye.

- The opposite (non-thrusting) hand has to participate in order for this technique to be successful.

- A helpful hint: Just after introduction of all of the additional components and just prior to applying the thrust, abduct the index finger into the segment you are moving.

7.3.2: Mid-cervical Spine Upslope – Chin Hold

Description: This is essentially the same technique as the previous one, except that the therapist uses a different hold. The patient is supine with their head on a pillow. The therapist grasps the patient, gently applying the proximal phalanx of their second finger to the lamina behind the transverse process of the affected segment. The opposite hand is wrapped around the chin and the patient's head is tucked between the therapist's lateral pectoral and anterior deltoid area. Contralateral rotation is introduced, followed by secondary levers of ipsilateral side-bending and slight extension prior to the thrust. Other levers are added as needed to engage the barrier further. This is also a two-handed technique in which the non-thrusting hand is critical for speed and control. The thrusting hand moves the patient into the primary lever of rotation while the opposite hand and arm assist with rotation by moving into the pillow simultaneously.

When to use: Pain with rotation and/or side-bending to the same side, or loss of unilateral rotation and side-bending to the same side.

Primary muscles activated: Elbow flexors, shoulder adductors and elevators on the thrusting side. Forearm supinators, shoulder adductors and depressors of the non-thrusting arm.

Suggested tests prior to thrust:
- AROM.
- Quadrant tests.
- Compression/traction tests.
- PPIVMs/PAIVMs.
- Shear tests.
- Pre-manipulative hold.

Patient position (Figure 7.3.2a)**:**
- Supine with head on a pillow.

Therapist position (Figure 7.3.2b)**:**
- Standing either to the side of the patient's head or at a 45-degree angle to the patient's head on the thrusting side.

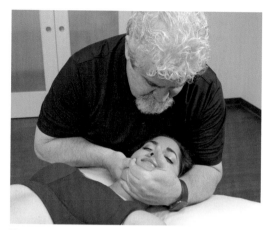

Figure 7.3.2a: Patient is supine with head on a pillow.

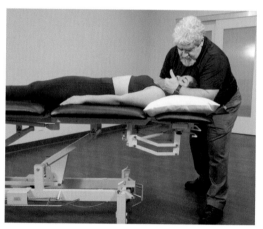

Figure 7.3.2b: Therapist stands to the side of the patient's head or at a 45 degree angle to the patient's head on the side to be thrusted.

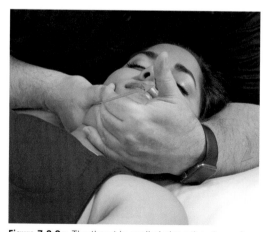

Figure 7.3.2c: The thrust is applied along the plane of the facet joint and into rotation.

Contacts points:
- The therapist's proximal phalanx of the second finger contacts the lamina behind the transverse process of the superior segment.

- The opposite hand reaches around and contacts the chin, while the corner of the patient's head rests in the area between the lateral pectorals and anterior deltoid. The therapist's same forearm rests on the side of the patient's head and face just anterior to the ear.

Position for the thrust:
- Primary lever of contralateral rotation is introduced until you feel the lamina of the superior segment come into your proximal phalanx of the thrusting hand.

- Ipsilateral side-bending to the level is then followed by adding slight extension.

- Translation, traction, additional compressions, vertically and horizontally, may be added to engage the barrier further.

Application of the thrust (Figure 7.3.2c)**:**
- The thrust is applied along the plane of the facet joint and into rotation.

- The opposite arm drops into the pillow at the same time.

Fine-tuning and keys to success:
- It is important to have the patient's head resting on a pillow to minimize tension in the neck that often occurs when lifting the head or having the head completely off the table.

- Have patient get as close to the top of the table as possible. This allows the therapist to add vertical compression with their trunk.

- Table should be at a level where the therapist can handle patient's head without much bend in their elbows when they are standing erect.

- Make sure your contact on the segment to be moved is back on the lamina of the superior segment.

- It is critical to have the patient's head tucked into the pocket between the lateral pectoral and anterior deltoid.

- Contact is further made with your non-thrusting forearm primarily. Compressing the patient's head into your chest allows better control.

- The hand on the chin is only resting around the chin and is not used to apply additional force or leverage.

- It is important not to lock down to the joint but to accumulate tension at the desired level.

- It is our experience that if you are getting too much activation of the sternocleidomastoid muscle on the thrust side, then you have introduced too much rotation as your primary lever.

- A good way to start rotation is to allow the head to fall into rotation onto the non-thrusting arm.

- Compression of the patient's head into your chest is critical prior to initiating this technique. The thrust is not initiated through the chin but with the thrusting hand and opposite forearm.

- Because this is an upslope technique, it is critical that this is a rotation around the vertex of the head toward the opposite eye.

- The opposite (non-thrusting) forearm has to participate in order for this technique to be successful.

- A helpful hint: Just after introduction of all of the additional components and just prior to applying the thrust, abduct the index finger into the segment you are moving.

7.3.3: Mid-cervical Spine Downslope – Cradle Hold

Description: This is a technique that uses side-bending as the primary lever. It is a two-hand technique in which the non-thrusting hand is critical for speed and control. The patient is supine with their head on a pillow. The therapist applies the proximal phalanx of their index finger onto the most lateral portion of the lamina of the affected segment. A primary lever of ipsilateral side-bending is introduced, followed by contralateral rotation and slight extension. Other levers such as translation, longitudinal compression and traction, etc. may be added. The non-thrusting hand is placed on the other side of the head. A thrust into a small amount of side-bending is applied once the barrier is fully engaged with the addition of the other levers. The direction of the thrust should be toward the patient's opposite axilla. The thrusting hand moves the patient into the primary lever of side-bending while the opposite hand assists by moving the head into side-bending simultaneously.

When to use: Pain with rotation and/or side-bending to the same side, or loss of unilateral rotation and side-bending to the same side.

Primary muscles activated: Shoulder flexors on the thrusting side. Shoulder extensors of the non-thrusting arm.

Suggested tests prior to thrust:
- AROM.
- Quadrant tests.
- Compression/traction tests.
- PPIVMs/PAIVMs.
- Shear tests.
- Pre-manipulative hold.

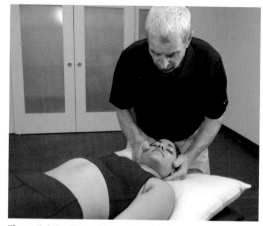

Figure 7.3.3a: Patient is supine with head on pillow and therapist stands at the head of the table on the thrusting side.

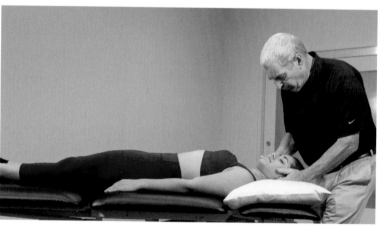

Figure 7.3.3b: Therapist takes up cradle hold.

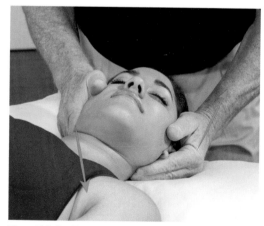

Figure 7.3.3c: Thrust is directed toward the patient's opposite axilla and applied downward along the plane of the facet joint and into side-bending.

Patient position (Figure 7.3.3a):
- Supine with head on a pillow.

Therapist position (Figure 7.3.3a):
- Standing at head of table on the thrusting side.

Contacts points:
- Proximal phalanx of second finger contacts the lateral aspect of the lamina just behind the transverse process of the superior segment.

- The opposite hand moves to the side of the head. The therapist's web space should be just behind the patient's ear.

Position for the thrust:
- Primary lever of ipsilateral side-bending is introduced until you feel the lamina of the superior segment come into your proximal phalanx of the thrusting hand.

- Contralateral rotation to the level is then followed by adding slight extension.

- Translation, traction, additional compressions, vertically and horizontally, may be added to engage the barrier further.

Application of the thrust (Figure 7.3.3c):
- The thrust is applied downward along the plane of the facet joint and into side-bending. The therapist should aim toward an area between the patient's sternum and opposite axilla.

- The opposite hand is pulled into the therapist's chest simultaneously.

Fine-tuning and keys to success:
- It is important to have the patient's head resting on a pillow to minimize tension in the neck that often occurs when lifting the head or having the head completely off the table.

- Have the patient get as close to the top of the table as possible. This allows the therapist to add vertical compression with their trunk.

- The table should be at a level where the therapist can handle the patient's head without much bend in their elbows when they are standing erect.

- Make sure your contact on the segment to be moved is as far lateral as possible on the lamina of the superior segment.

- Keep the non-thrusting hand up along the side of the skull above the ear for better control with this technique.

- Caution must be used with excessive side-bending and/or translation as it places too much stress on the contralateral tissues and can cause injury to your patient.

- The opposite (non-thrusting) hand has to participate in order for this technique to be successful.

- It is critical that the non-thrusting hand is pulled toward your chest to form an axis of motion around the nose and generate the appropriate speed.

- A helpful hint: Just after introduction of all of the additional components and just prior to applying the thrust, abduct the index finger into the segment you are moving.

7.3.4: Mid-cervical Spine Downslope – Chin Hold

Description: This is essentially the same technique as the previous one, except that the therapist uses a different hold. The patient is supine with their head on a pillow. The therapist grasps the patient, gently applying the proximal phalanx of their second finger to the lamina as far lateral as possible and behind the transverse process of the affected segment. The opposite hand is wrapped around the chin and the patient's head is tucked between the therapist's lateral pectoral and anterior deltoid area. Ipsilateral side-bending is introduced, followed by secondary levers of contralateral rotation and slight extension prior to the thrust. Other levers are added as needed to engage the barrier further. This is also a two-handed technique in which the non-thrusting forearm and hand is critical for speed and control. The thrusting hand moves the patient into the primary lever of side-bending while the opposite hand and arm assist with side-bending by moving toward the therapist's chest simultaneously.

When to use: Pain with rotation and/or side-bending to the same side, or loss of unilateral rotation and side-bending to the same side.

Primary muscles activated: Shoulder flexors on the thrusting side. Shoulder extensors of the non-thrusting arm.

Suggested tests prior to thrust:
- AROM.
- Quadrant tests.
- Compression/traction tests.
- PPIVMs/PAIVMs.
- Shear tests.
- Pre-manipulative hold.

Patient position (Figure 7.3.4a)**:**
- Supine with head resting on a pillow.

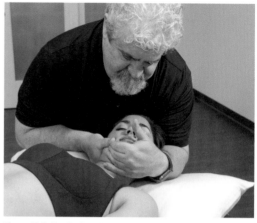
Figure 7.3.4a: Patient is supine with head on pillow and therapist stands at the head of the table on the thrusting side.

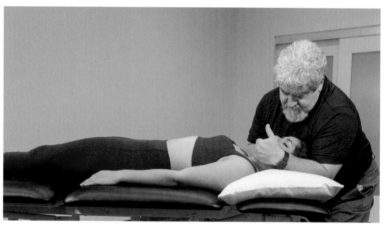
Figure 7.3.4b: Therapist takes up chin hold.

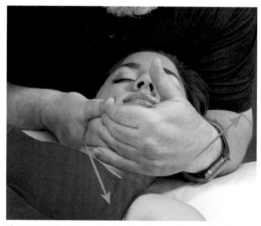
Figure 7.3.4c: Thrust is directed toward the patient's opposite axilla and applied downward along the plane of the facet joint and into side-bending.

Therapist position (Figure 7.3.4b):
- Standing either to the side of the patient's head or at a 45-degree angle to the patient's head on the thrusting side.

Contacts points:
- Proximal phalanx of second finger contacts the lateral aspect of the lamina just behind the transverse process of the superior segment.

- The opposite hand reaches around and contacts the chin while the corner of the patient's head rests in the area between the lateral pectorals and anterior deltoid. The therapist's same forearm rests on the side of the patient's head and face just anterior to the ear.

Position for the thrust:
- Primary lever of ipsilateral side-bending is introduced until you feel the lamina of the superior segment come into your proximal phalanx of the thrusting hand.

- Contralateral rotation to the level is then followed by adding slight extension.

- Translation, traction, additional compressions, vertically and horizontally, may be added to engage the barrier further.

Application of the thrust (Figure 7.3.4c):
- The thrust is applied downward along the plane of the facet joint and into side-bending. The therapist should aim toward an area between the patient's sternum and opposite axilla.

- The opposite arm and hand is pulled into the therapist's chest simultaneously.

Fine-tuning and keys to success:
- It is important to have the patient's head resting on a pillow to minimize tension in the neck that often occurs when lifting the head or having the head completely off the table.

- Have patient get as close to the top of the table as possible. This allows the therapist to add vertical compression with their trunk.

- Table should be at a level where the therapist can handle patient's head without excessive amount of forward bending of their trunk.

- Make sure your contact on the segment to be moved is as far lateral as possible on the lamina of the superior segment.

- It is critical to have the patient's head tucked into the pocket between the therapist's lateral pectorals and anterior deltoid.

- Contact is further made with the non-thrusting forearm primarily. Compressing the patient's head into your chest allows better control.

- The hand on the chin is only resting around the chin and is not used to apply additional force or leverage.

- The opposite (non-thrusting) forearm has to participate in order for this technique to be successful.

- It is critical that the non-thrusting hand is pulled toward your chest to form an axis of motion around the nose and generate the appropriate speed.

- A helpful hint: Just after introduction of all of the additional components and just prior to applying the thrust, abduct the index finger into the segment you are moving.

7.3.5: Supine Cervical Spine Traction Thrust

Description: This technique can use either side-bending or rotation as the initial lever for positioning purposes only. The MCP or proximal phalanx of second finger is placed on the lamina of the segment to be moved. Ipsilateral side-bending followed by contralateral rotation and extension are added to allow for a better purchase on the affected segment. Adding additional components as needed, the thrust is applied in straight cephalic direction.

When to use: Good technique in the presence of certain radicular symptoms and in conditions where rotary and translatory techniques are too aggressive or there is high irritability. Should not be used when you suspect an instability or hypermobility either at or adjacent to the joint.

Primary muscles activated: Shoulder adductors of thrusting hand and shoulder abductors of opposite hand.

Suggested tests prior to thrust:
- AROM.
- Quadrant testing.
- Sheer testing.
- PPIVMs/PAIVMs.
- Traction/compression.
- Pre-manipulative hold.

Patient position (Figure 7.3.5a):
- Supine with head on a pillow.

Therapist position (Figure 7.3.5a):
- Standing at the side of the table at the patient's head.

Contact points:
- MCP/proximal phalanx of second finger of thrusting hand contacts lamina of segment to be moved.

- The opposite hand assumes the chin hold with the forearm resting on the side of the patient's skull.

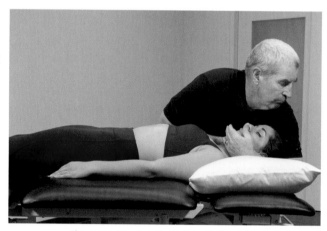

Figure 7.3.5a: Patient supine with head on a pillow and therapist stands at the side of the table at the patient's head.

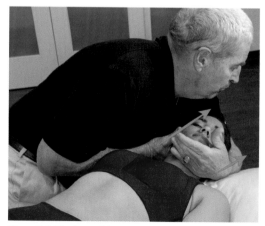

Figure 7.3.5b: A small impulse is applied toward the vertex of the patient's head producing a traction-like force at the contact point.

Position for the thrust:
- Ipsilateral side-bending with contralateral rotation followed by slight extension and compression at the level are introduced.

Application of the thrust (Figure 7.3.5b)**:**
- Slack is taken up once the various levers are introduced.

- A small impulse is applied toward the vertex of the head producing a traction-like force.

Fine tuning and keys to success:
- It is helpful to have the patient lie diagonally on the table so that the head is close to the therapist for easier handling.

- Table should be set at a height just below the therapist's iliac crests.

- The therapist should align himself or herself so that their body lines up in a cephalic position relative to the patient.

- Foot on the side of the thrusting hand should be back.

- Be careful to make light contact around the chin as increased tension can cause potential problems with the TMJ.

- Most of the traction force is being applied through the thrusting hand and opposite forearm.

- You should apply a mild traction to the segment prior to the thrust.

- Traction is applied with the thrusting hand and the opposite forearm and not through the chin.

- When applying thrust force, it should be a small enough impulse so as not to move the entire body.

- Try to use your body to help with applying the thrust for better force and amplitude control.

7.4: Cervicothoracic Junction

7.4.1: Prone CT Junction Lateral Flexion Thrust

Description: This is a prone technique where the patient faces away from the therapist. The patient rests their head on their orbit while their hand farthest from the therapist rests at the end of the table above their head. Have them look up at their hand. The other hand is at their side. The therapist takes up the hand hold by applying the proximal phalanx of the second finger to tissues abutting C7. The opposite hand reaches around and contacts the zygomatic arch cupping around but not on the patient's ear. Slack is taken up in opposite directions with both hands and a thrust is applied to C7 on T1 into lateral flexion toward the patient's opposite axilla.

When to use: This is a good technique to apply with a CT unilateral dysfunction. It can be used down to T2-3 depending on the morphology of the patient. It is much more challenging on the heavier patient and those with excessive thoracic kyphosis.

Primary muscles activated: Shoulder flexors of thrusting hand and shoulder adductors of non-thrusting hand.

Suggested tests prior to thrust:
- Johnston Tap Test.
- AROM.
- Palpation of landmarks.
- PPIVMS/PAIVMs.
- Quadrant testing.

Patient position (Figure 7.4.1a):
- Patient is prone near the edge of the table.

- The patient's far hand reaches up at or above the head level and rests on the table.

- The near hand is at their side.

- The patient's head is resting on their orbit looking away from the therapist.

Therapist position (Figure 7.4.1a):
- Standing to the side of the patient below their shoulder.

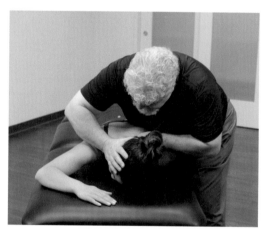

Figure 7.4.1a: Patient is prone near the edge of the table with right arm elevated and resting on left orbit.

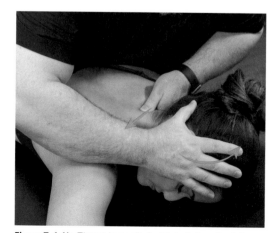

Figure 7.4.1b: Thrust is applied with both hands – left hand toward patient's axilla and right hand introducing lower cervical lateral flexion.

Contact points:

- Contact by the therapist is a pincer grip, with the thumb lateral to the spinous process of C7 and the proximal phalanx of the second finger on the tissues immediately adjacent to C7 spinous process.

- The opposite hand contacts the patient's zygomatic arch.

Position for the thrust:

- The therapist begins by moving C7 with their thrusting hand to take up the slack until the head begins to rotate.

- With the opposite hand, through the zygomatic arch move the head/neck into rotation and side-bending with slight extension until you engage the barrier.

Application of thrust (Figure 7.4.1b):

- After gathering all of the forces with both hands, the primary thrust is toward the patient's opposite axilla.

- The opposite hand provides the counterforce into opposite direction through the head.

Fine-tuning and keys to success:

- An easy way to get the patient to position their head properly is to have them look up at their hand on that side while they rest on their orbit.

- The table should be set just below waist level to make easy access to the patient possible and to guarantee better success.

- The therapist needs to place one foot back with the technique to improve leverage.

- It is critical that the thrusting hand not make sole contact with the spinous process of C7. This can be quite uncomfortable.

- The pincer grip is essential to the success of this technique (see Figure 7.4.1c).

- Avoid putting your hand over the patient's ear. Contact should be on the zygomatic arch with the web space of the thumb and index finger going around the ear.

- We have found that resting your non-thrusting hand on the patient's upper thorax and/or shoulder places it in the optimal position to contact the patient's head.

- The amount of force into extension and side-bending with the non-thrusting hand is minimal when counter pressure is applied to engage the barrier. The head will naturally fall into slight side-bending and extension when the counterforce is applied.

- It is helpful to activate your core and use your body and legs along with your thrusting hand to accomplish the thrust. This seems to allow the therapist the best control when applying the thrust.

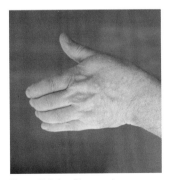

Figure 7.4.1c: Pincer grip.

7.4.2: Seated CT Junction Rotatory Thrust

Description: This is a seated technique to restore rotation of C7 on T1. The following description is for treatment to the left C7/T1. The patient is seated on a low stool and the therapist stands behind the patient's right shoulder. The patient's left shoulder is prepositioned into posterior rotation by retracting it so that the left hand falls behind the patient. The therapist places their left hand so that the thumb contacts the lateral side of the T1 spinous process, and the fingers lightly grasp the left clavicle. This will cause left rotation at T1 relative to C7. The therapist then places their right forearm across the patient's left side of the face and ulnar border of the right hand directly above their left hand at C7. The thrust is provided along the plane of the CT junction with the both hands into rotation. This two-handed technique allows good control and is a good alternative to the prone technique, especially for larger individuals and those with increased CT kyphosis.

When to use: When there is loss of rotation to one side at the CT junction.

Primary muscles activated: Shoulder abductors and retractors of both arms.

Suggested tests prior to thrust:
- Johnston tap test.
- AROM.
- Palpation of landmarks.
- PPIVMS/PAIVMs.
- Quadrant testing.

Patient position (Figure 7.4.2a)**:**
- Seated on low stool.

Therapist position (Figure 7.4.2a)**:**
- Standing behind the patient on the opposite side to that being treated.

Contact points:
- Therapist contacts patient's right shoulder with their anterior hip/trunk. This provides some compression and movement control using the therapist's body.

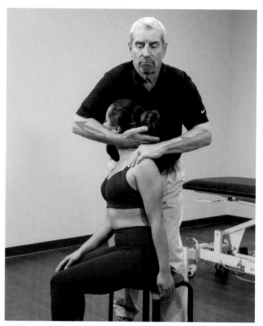

Figure 7.4.2a: Patient seated on low stool and therapist standing behind the patient's opposite shoulder (in this case right). Patient's ipsilateral shoulder is prepositioned back to produce rotation from below.

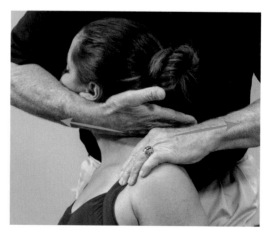

Figure 7.4.2b: Thrust is achieved by rapid abduction of both arms causing right rotation at C7 with the ulnar border of the right hand and left hand providing counterforce on T1 into left rotation.

- The patient's left shoulder is gripped as the therapist's four fingers of the left hand reaches over the left clavicle while the left thumb rests just lateral to the spinous process of T1.

- Contact with the lamina of C7 on the left side is made with the ulnar border of the therapist's right hand.

Position for the thrust:
- The therapist continues to move their hip into the patient's right shoulder to increase compression and control.

- The patient's left shoulder is dropped and placed in a retracted position producing relative left rotation at T1.

- Left side-bending is introduced, followed by right rotation, followed by either slight flexion or extension.

- Traction may be introduced at the end to further engage the barrier.

Application of thrust (Figure 7.4.2b)**:**
- After gathering all of the forces, the thrust is directed into right rotation at C7 with the right hand by pulling the patient's head and neck in a direction toward the therapist's body.

- The left hand provides the counterforce on T1 into left rotation.

Fine-tuning and keys to success:
- The patient should sit so their shoulder is level with the therapist's abdomen.

- The forearm of the therapist's top hand makes contact along the side of the patient's skull just above the ear.

- The ulnar border of the therapist's top hand is on the lamina of C7.

- Avoid pronating the top hand and reaching around the skull as it adds too much of a lever and can potentially harm your patient.

- It is vital that the palm of the top hand be open and faces the ceiling, i.e. supinated.

- Keep the top hand as close to the bottom hand as possible so as to get a precise movement at this joint.

- Compressing the patient toward you using your hip against the right shoulder allows you to circumduct and side-bend the patient with your body.

- Excessive rotation of the head and neck is prevented by the therapist's trunk.

- The contact is such that when the therapist leans backward, left side-bending is introduced.

- The addition of traction and circumduction allow you to engage the barrier better just prior to application of the thrust.

7.4.3: Seated CT Junction Traction with Arm-hold Variation

Description: This is a seated technique whereby the therapist applies traction to the CT junction. The patient is seated at the edge of the table with the therapist behind them. The therapist grabs the patient's wrists as the patient interlocks their fingers over their CT junction. The force is focused over the CT junction by having the patient pronate their hands and wrists as the therapist provides a traction force through the patient's axilla and wrists. Additional components of side-bending and rotation with the patient breathing out can be added to improve focusing. The traction thrust is directed up and back.

When to use: When there is a bilateral or unilateral fixation of C7 on T1.

Primary muscles activated: Shoulder flexors and elevators actively contract with simultaneous contraction of the therapist's quads into extension.

Suggested tests prior to thrust:
- PPIVMs/PAIVMs.
- AROM.
- Quadrant testing.
- Palpation of landmarks.
- Johnston tap test.

Patient position (Figure 7.4.3a)**:**
- Seated on table with buttocks close to its edge.

Therapist position (Figure 7.4.3a)**:**
- Standing close to the table with one leg back directly behind the patient.

Contact points:
- Therapist intertwines arms through the patient's and grabs both wrists.

- Therapists forearms should be tucked in to the patient's axillae.

- Contact is also made with the therapist's sternum on the upper T spine of the patient.

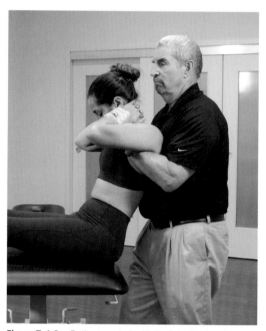

Figure 7.4.3a: Patient seated with both buttocks close to edge and therapist standing behind patient with one leg back.

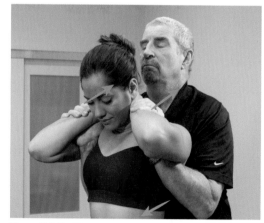

Figure 7.4.3b: Thrust is a traction force by the therapist with their forearms and body through patient's axillae.

Position for the thrust:
- Patient is gently flexed and extended to the level of the CT junction by the therapist using their arms and chest.

- Additional components of side-bending and rotation in opposite directions can be added as the patient breathes out.

Application of the thrust (Figure 7.4.3b)**:**
- Thrust is accomplished by applying traction with the therapist leaning back. The actual force is applied from the legs attempting to straighten at the knees while lifting through the patient's axilla and arms.

Fine tuning and keys to success:
- Patient can be in a long sit position or with their legs folded on the table.

- They should be as close to the edge of the table as possible.

- The table height should be set so that the patient's shoulders line up with the therapist's clavicles when they are standing completely upright.

- When the therapist engages contact with the patient with one leg back, this places them in the optimal position to accomplish the thrust.

- If you can have the patient interlock their hands so as to have both index fingers resting over the CT junction, focusing and localization will be better.

- The therapist must keep their knees slightly flexed and use their chest as a fulcrum over the CT junction to localize the forces.

- It is the active contraction of the shoulder elevators that are critical to the success of this technique.

- The slack is taken up prior to the technique with the therapist pulling up and back toward them.

- Side-bending and rotation in opposite directions may be added just before thrusting.

- Speed is critical here. Try to apply the impulse as quickly as possible with minimal to no buttock lift off the table.

- It often works better if you ask the patient to breathe out as you thrust.

7.4.4: Seated CT Junction Traction with Neck-hold Variation

Description: This technique is a seated technique whereby the therapist applies traction to the CT junction. This is a variation of the arm hold where the therapist makes actual contact at the CT junction interlocking their hands. In this case, the patient's hands are placed over the therapist's hands. Localization is sought with the therapist's chest with varying degrees of flexion and extension. Additional components of side-bending and rotation along with having the patient breathe out may be added to enhance focusing. The clinician's hands are pronated as traction is applied upward and backward at the CT junction.

When to use: When there is a bilateral or unilateral fixation of C7 on T1.

Primary muscles activated: Shoulder flexors and elevators actively contract with simultaneous contraction of the therapist's quads into extension.

Suggested tests prior to thrust:
- PPIVMs/PAIVMs.
- AROM.
- Quadrant testing.
- Palpation of landmarks.
- Johnston tap test.

Patient position (Figure 7.4.4a)**:**
- Seated on table with buttocks close to its edge.

Therapist position (Figure 7.4.4b)**:**
- Standing close to the table with one leg back directly behind the patient.

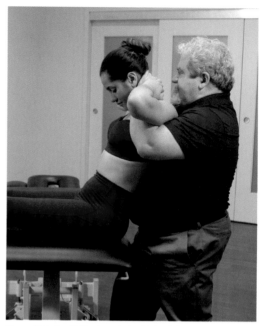

Figure 7.4.4a: Patient seated with both buttocks close to edge and therapist standing behind patient with one leg back.

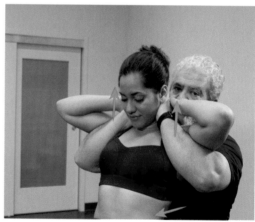

Figure 7.4.4b: Thrust is a traction force by the therapist with their forearms and body through patient's axillae.

Contact points:
- Therapist intertwines arms through the patient's and hands are placed at the CT junction.

- Therapists forearms should be tucked in to the patient's axilla.

- Contact is also made with the therapist's sternum on the upper T spine of the patient.

Position for the thrust:
- Patient is gently flexed and extended at the CT junction by the therapist using their chest.

- Some side-bending and rotation in opposite directions can be added for further focusing if needed.

Application of the thrust (Figure 7.4.4b)**:**
- Thrust is accomplished by applying traction with the therapist leaning back.

- The actual force is applied from the legs attempting to straighten at the knees while lifting through the CT junction and upper T spine.

Fine tuning and keys to success:
- Patient can be in a long sit position or with their legs folded on the table.

- They should be as close to the edge of the table as possible.

- The table height should be set so that the patient's shoulders line up with the therapist's clavicles when they are standing completely upright.

- When the therapist engages contact with the patient with one leg back this places them in the optimal position to accomplish the thrust.

- The therapist's wrists should be almost fully extended and forearms should be pronated to allow a better purchase of the joint prior to thrusting.

- Try to position your crossed hands so that both index fingers are superimposed over the CT junction for precise localization.

- The therapist must keep their knees slightly flexed and use their chest as a fulcrum over the CT junction.

- The slack is taken up prior to the technique with the therapist pulling upward and backward toward them.

- Speed is critical here. Try to apply the impulse as quickly as possible with minimal to no buttock lift off the table.

- Having the patient breathe out just before the thrust also seems to improve the success of this technique.

- It is the active contraction of the shoulder elevators that are the most critical to the success of this technique.

7.5: Thoracic Spine

7.5.1: Supine Mid Thoracic Facet Thrust

Description: This is a supine mid thoracic thrust also known as the "dog" technique. The patient is placed in the supine position with arms folded over each other. The therapist places their bottom hand over the affected segment. The therapist can contact the affected segment using a pistol grip, fist grip, or palmar grip (see Figure 7.5.1a). The therapist contacts the patient's forearms with the forearm of their thrusting or upper hand. After the therapist locates the affected segment with their bottom hand, caudal traction is applied with it. The therapist adds additional levers of ipsilateral side-bending and contralateral rotation to the thorax to further engage the barrier. This will only result in a small amount of movement at the segment. Immediately prior to the thrust, the lower hand is pronated while, simultaneously, the therapist's bottom forearm adducts against the lateral trunk as the wrist and hand is pronated at the segment.

When to use: This can be used to restore unilateral loss of side-bending and rotation to the same side at a segment or bilateral facet involvement.

Primary muscles activated: Shoulder protractors of thrusting arm. Forearm pronators and shoulder adductors on the opposite side.

Suggested tests prior to thrust:
- Johnston Tap test.
- Palpation for pain and position.
- Quadrant testing to the thoracic spine.
- Seated inspiration with both thoracic flexion. and extension to incriminate pain.
- Axial thoracic compression and traction.

Patient position (Figure 7.5.1b)**:**
- Supine on table with head on pillow. Arms are folded elbow to elbow, usually with the far arm on top.

Therapist position (Figure 7.5.1b)**:**
- Standing to the side of the table at the patient's mid thorax, facing toward their head.

Contact points (Figure 7.5.1b)**:**
- For bilateral lesions, the therapist contacts bilateral transverse processes at the affected level.

- For unilateral lesions, the therapist contacts the ipsilateral transverse process above and the contralateral transverse process of lower segment.

- The forearm of the therapist's thrusting hand contacts the folded arms of the patient.

Position for the thrust:
- The patient is moved toward the therapist.

- The therapist's bottom hand tractions caudally at the segment.

- The therapist initially adds compression through the patient's arms into their thorax, followed by side-bending, then rotation.

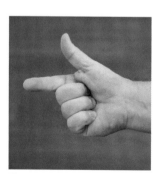

Figure 7.5.1a: Pistol grip

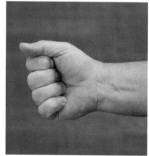

Fist grip

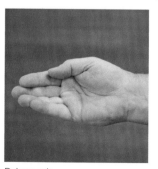

Palmar grip

- The forearm of the thrusting hand takes up slack through the patient's chest and arms in a cephalic direction to engage the barrier prior to the thrust.

- The therapist's bottom hand will pronate as the rotation from in front is introduced into it. This hand will radial deviate as contralateral side-bending is introduced.

Application of the thrust (Figure 7.5.1c):
- Thrust is applied through the patient's arms into the table directed toward the patient's head.

- Two things occur simultaneously with the thrust. The therapist adducts their forearm into the patient's lateral thorax, and they pronate the same forearm and hand at the affected segment.

Fine-tuning and keys to success:
- It is helpful to place the patient four to six inches or a fist width from the edge of the table for consistent positioning for each treatment.

- The therapist should stand facing the patient's opposite shoulder with the foot back on the side of the thrusting hand.

- Of the three contact grip options, the palmar grip seems to be most comfortable to the patient and therapist alike.

- The therapist should stay as upright as possible through their trunk to maintain their core, enabling them to take up the slack from above and below the patient's trunk. Keeping the head up will also help.

- It is very helpful for the therapist to tighten their interscapular muscles by adducting the scapulae to get further engagement of the barrier prior to the thrust. This will also help with tightening the core.

- It is the movement of the therapist's body that introduces the various levers/components rather than their hand and forearm.

- After the patient is in a position ready to thrust, additional components may be needed to achieve the best "focus" for the thrust. The therapist can further test the barrier by having the patient rotate the neck and/or move the eyes in different directions.

- Most essential is timing the thrust with the pronation of the lower hand at the moment of thrust.

- The direction of the thrust is into the table and toward the patient's head. Do not apply the thrust directly into the patient's shoulder joints.

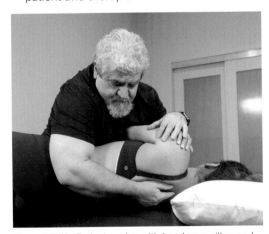

Figure 7.5.1b: Patient supine with head on a pillow and arms folded elbow to elbow, and therapist standing to side of table at patient's mid thorax.

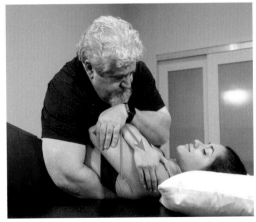

Figure 7.5.1c: Thrust is applied through the patient's arms into the table and directed toward the patient's head.

7.5.2: Supine Upper Thoracic Spine Thrust

Description: This is a technique that allows the therapist to thrust the upper T spine in the supine position. The patient is placed supine on the table with their hands behind their neck and their elbows close together. This allows the therapist to leverage and locate the segment through the arms. The larger patient can also be placed with their arms crossed over the top of each other. The therapist contacts the patient's arms with their thrusting forearm. The bottom hand contacts the affected segment with their thenar eminence using a fist or palmar contact. The patient is flexed to the level. Additional components of side-bending, rotation, and other levers can be added to further engage the barrier. The thrust is applied through compression into the table in a cephalic direction.

When to use: This can be used with patients with dysfunctions in the top second through fifth thoracic vertebrae. It has been our experience that this technique is not as optimum with heavier patients and those with increased upper thoracic kyphosis.

Major muscles activated: Shoulder depressors of thrusting hand side. Forearm pronators of non-thrusting hand in conjunction with the body drop.

Suggested tests prior to thrust:
- Johnston Tap Test.
- Palpation for pain and position.
- Quadrant testing to the thoracic spine.
- Seated inspiration with both upper thoracic. flexion and extension to incriminate pain.
- Axial thoracic compression and traction.
- PPIVMs/PAIVMs.

Patient position (Figure 7.5.2b)**:**
- Supine on table with head on pillow.

- The patient's hands are placed behind their neck.

- Their elbows are placed together making them easier to handle.

Therapist position (Figure 7.5.2b)**:**
- Standing to the side of the table at the patient's mid to upper thorax facing toward the patient's head.

Contact points (Figure 7.5.2a)**:**
- For bilateral lesions, the therapist contacts bilateral transverse processes at the affected level.

- For unilateral lesions, the therapist contacts the ipsilateral transverse process above and the contralateral transverse process of lower segment.

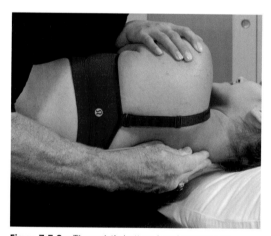

Figure 7.5.2a: Therapist's bottom hand tractions the affected segment caudally toward the patient's feet.

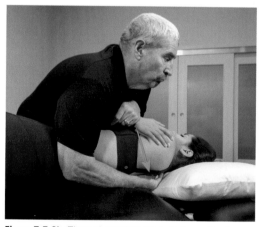

Figure 7.5.2b: Thrust is applied through the patient's forearms into the table directed toward their head.

- The forearm of the thrusting hand contacts the folded elbows of the patient.

- Lower hand is held in a loose fist over the affected segment(s).

Position for the thrust:
- Patient is moved toward the therapist.

- The therapist's bottom hand tractions the affected segment caudally toward the patient's feet.

- The therapist initially adds compression through the patient's arms, followed by side-bending, then rotation with the thrusting arm if needed.

- The forearm of the therapist's thrusting hand takes up slack through the patient's forearms in a cephalic direction to engage the barrier prior to the thrust.

- The therapist's bottom hand will pronate as rotation is introduced with the thrusting hand above. Simultaneously, the lower hand will radially deviate as contralateral side-bending is introduced from the thrusting hand above.

Application of the thrust (Figure 7.5.2b):
- The thrust is applied through the patient's forearms into the table directed toward their head.

- The lower hand simultaneously pronates as the same forearm adducts into the patient's thorax.

Fine-tuning and keys to success:
- It is helpful to place the patient four to six inches or a fist width from the edge of the table for consistent positioning for each treatment.

- Flexing the patient's opposite knee when rolling the patient makes it easier to roll a patient toward you, especially with larger individuals.

- Stand facing the patient's opposite shoulder with your foot back on the side of your thrusting hand.

- The table should be higher than mid-thigh.

- Of the three thoracic contact grip options, the palmar grip seems to be most comfortable for the patient and therapist alike.

- The therapist should stay as upright as possible through their trunk to maintain their core, enabling them to take up the slack from above and below the patient's trunk. Keeping the head up will also help.

- It is very helpful to tighten your interscapular muscles by adducting the scapulae to get further engagement of the barrier prior to the thrust. This will also help with tightening your core.

- After the patient is in a position ready to thrust, additional components may be needed to achieve the best "focus" for the thrust.

- The best way to maintain an upright posture throughout the thrust is to keep your head up.

- Most essential is timing the thrust with the pronation of your bottom hand at the moment of thrust.

- The direction of the thrust is into the table and toward the patient's head. Do not apply the thrust directly into the patient's shoulder joints.

- Timing by having the patient breathe out during the thrust and different positioning of the legs in flexion and/or extension can also make a difference in better engaging the barrier for a more successful application of the thrust.

7.5.3: Supine Lower Thoracic Spine Thrust

Description: The patient is placed in the supine position with their arms folded over each other. The therapist rolls the patient toward them so as to be able to make contact with the affected segment with the lower hand using a palmar grip. The therapist applies a traction force in a cephalic direction with that hand to encourage flexion. The top forearm of the thrusting hand makes contact with the patient's forearms. The patient is flexed to the level of the affected segment. The therapist adds ipsilateral side-bending and contralateral rotation to further engage the barrier. The thrust is made directing the force in a posterior and superior direction through the patient's forearms. The therapist produces simultaneous forearm adduction into the trunk and hand pronation with the non-thrusting hand into the segment.

When to use: This can be used to restore unilateral loss of side-bending and rotation to the same side at a segment or bilateral facet involvement.

Primary muscles activated: Shoulder protractors and depressors of thrusting arm. Forearm pronators and shoulder adductors on the opposite side.

Suggested tests prior to thrust:
- Johnston Tap Test.
- Palpation for pain and position.
- PPIVMS/PAIVMS.
- Seated inspiration with both thoracic flexion and extension to incriminate pain.
- Axial thoracic compression and traction.

Patient position (Figure 7.5.3b):
- Supine on table with head on pillow. Arms are folded elbow to elbow, usually with the far arm on top.

Therapist position (Figure 7.5.3b):
- Standing to the side of the table at the patient's mid thorax facing toward the patient's head.

Contact points (Figure 7.5.3a):
- For bilateral lesions, the therapist contacts bilateral transverse processes at the affected level.

- For unilateral lesions, the therapist contacts the ipsilateral transverse process above and the contralateral transverse process of lower segment.

- The forearm of the thrusting hand contacts the folded arms of the patient.

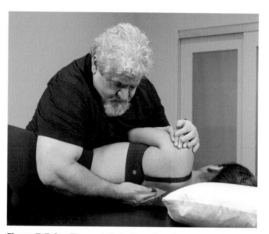

Figure 7.5.3a: Therapist's bottom hand contacts the affected segment and tractions the patient's spine in a cephalic direction.

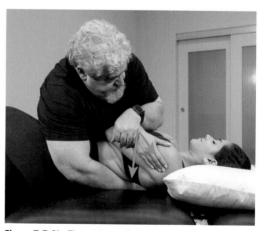

Figure 7.5.3b: Thrust is applied through the patient's forearms into the table directed toward the patient's head.

Position for the thrust:

- Patient is moved toward the therapist.

- The therapist's bottom hand contacts the affected segment and tractions the patient's spine in a cephalic direction.

- The therapist initially adds compression through the patient's arms, followed by side-bending, then rotation with the thrusting arm if needed.

- The therapist takes up slack through the patient's chest and arms in a cephalic direction with their thrusting forearm to further engage the barrier prior to the thrust.

- The therapist's bottom hand will pronate as rotation is introduced with the thrusting hand above. Simultaneously, the lower hand will radial deviate as contralateral side-bending is introduced from the thrusting hand above.

Application of the thrust (Figure 7.5.3b)**:**

- Thrust is applied through the patient's forearms into the table directed toward the patient head.

- The therapist's lower hand simultaneously pronates as the same forearm adducts into the patient's thorax simultaneously with the thrust.

Fine-tuning and keys to success:

- It is helpful to place the patient four to six inches or a fist width from the edge of the table for consistent positioning for each treatment.

- Flexing the patient's opposite knee when rolling the patient makes it easier to roll a patient toward you, especially with larger individuals.

- Stand facing the patient's opposite shoulder with your foot back on the side of the thrusting hand.

- The table should be higher than mid-thigh.

- Of the three thoracic contact grip options, the palmar grip seems to be most comfortable to patient and therapist alike.

- Stay as upright as possible through the trunk to maintain your core to take up the slack from atop and below the patient's trunk. Keeping your head up will help.

- It is very helpful to tighten your interscapular muscles by adducting the scapulae to get further engagement of the barrier prior to the thrust. This will also help with tightening your core.

- After the patient is in a position ready to thrust, additional components may be needed to achieve the best "focus" for the thrust.

- The best way to maintain an upright posture throughout the thrust is to keep your head up.

- Most essential is timing the thrust with the pronation of your bottom hand at the moment of thrust.

- Timing by having the patient breathe out during the thrust and different positioning of the legs in flexion and/or extension can also make a big difference, better engaging the barrier for a more successful application of the thrust.

- The direction of the thrust is into the table and toward the patient's head. Do not apply the thrust directly into the patient's shoulder joints.

7.5.4: Prone PA (Screw) Mid Thoracic Spine Thrust

Description: This is a prone technique where the patient can either rest their face in the hole in the treatment table (assuming there is one) or rest with their face toward their preferred side. The patient's arms can be adjusted to introduce some thoracic extension (arms up and hands under forehead) or to minimize thoracic extension (arms by the sides of the body). The arms can also be placed with elbows and forearms hanging from the treatment table as a sort of mid-range starting position. The therapist takes up the hand hold by applying the pisiform of each hand to the tissues overlying the costotransverse joints of the level to be treated. Slack is taken up by rotating the pisiform contacts in either a clockwise or counterclockwise direction. The thrust is applied in a posterior-to-anterior direction while also moving one hand in a cephalad direction and the other in a caudal direction.

When to use: This can be used to restore loss of mid thoracic extension, as well as loss of side-bending and rotation to one side at a segment or bilateral facet or costotransverse joint involvement.

Primary muscles activated: Shoulder adductors of both hands and trunk abdominals (core).

Suggested tests prior to thrust:
- Johnston Tap Test.
- Palpation for pain and position.
- Quadrant testing to the thoracic spine.
- Seated inspiration with both thoracic flexion and extension to incriminate pain.
- Axial thoracic compression and traction.

Patient position (Figure 7.5.4a)**:**
- Patient is prone near the edge of the table.

- The patient's face can rest in the face hole of the treatment table (assuming there is one) or can be turned to their preferred side.

- The therapist can apply the technique with slight variation in the thoracic extension by placing the patient's arms and hands up under their forehead to start in slightly more thoracic extension; or with the arms and hands at the side of the body to start in slightly less thoracic extension.

- The patient's starting position (arm placement) should be predicated on patient comfort.

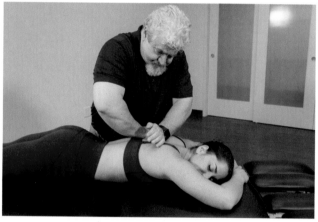

Figure 7.5.4a: Patient prone near edge of table and therapist stands directly over segment to be treated.

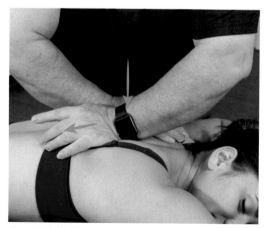

Figure 7.5.4b: Thrust is toward the table, with a simultaneous cephalad force with one hand and caudal force with the other.

Therapist position (Figure 7.5.4a)**:**
- Standing to the side of the table at the patient's mid thorax perpendicular to the patient's body.

Contact points:
- Contact by the therapist is through the pisiform and ulnar border of each hand.

- One pisiform contact is on the costotransverse joint of the level to be treated, and the other pisiform contact can be on the costotransverse joint on the opposite side; a) at the same level, b) one level above, or c) one level below.

Position for the thrust:
- The therapist begins by placing their pisiform contacts on the selected levels and rotates their contact points (either clockwise or counterclockwise) as they apply downward pressure (PA) toward the treatment table. The therapist's arms should be straight and the downward pressure should come from their body weight leaning onto the patient's thorax.

Application of thrust (Figure 7.5.4b)**:**
- After gathering all of the forces with both hands, the primary thrust is toward the treatment table, with a simultaneous cephalad force with one hand and caudal force with the other.

- The thrust onto the patient's thorax should be through a very small amplitude.

Fine-tuning and keys to success:
- It is helpful to place the patient four to six inches or a fist width from the edge of the table for consistent positioning for each treatment.

- The table should be set just below waist level to make easy access to the patient possible and to guarantee better success.

- The therapist can take up a comfortable squat stance or place one foot back with the technique to improve leverage.

- It is critical that the thrust be applied through as short a range as possible to minimize risk of post-treatment soreness.

- Experienced clinicians and teachers will say that the ratio of PA thrust to cephalad/caudal thrust should be 60:40, and minimizing the PA component does add a level of safety in terms of avoiding excessive peak forces.

- It is permissible to let the patient fully exhale and hold prior to the thrust.

- It is helpful to activate your core and use your body and legs along with your thrusting hands to accomplish the thrust. This seems to allow the therapist the best control when applying the thrust.

7.5.5: Lateral Thoracic Thrust for Ring Lesion in Sidelying

Description: This is not a common technique but a very effective one for treating ring lesions first described by Canadian physiotherapist Diane Lee. The patient is initially placed supine with their arms folded over each other on the table. The therapist reaches across the patient's opposite side and firmly grasps the affected rib with a lumbrical grip. The therapist rolls the patient on to the hand gripping the affected rib. A short, quick thrust is applied into the bottom hand toward the table. It requires very little force. Hence, caution with amplitude is essential. Testing for this will involve translating the thoracic spine from side to side to assess movement. This involves a scooping motion.

When to use: This technique is used to treat thoracic rim lesions or loss of side-to-side shifting at a certain level. It is used when the treatment of typical thoracic dysfunctions is not responding to repeated thrust manipulations/mobilizations.

Primary muscles activated: Lumbricals of lower hand. Shoulder depressors of thrusting arm and trunk flexors.

Suggested tests prior to thrust:
- Quadrant testing in thoracic spine.
- Side-to-side translation through the rib cage.
- Johnston Tap Test.
- Palpation for pain and position.

Patient position (Figure 7.5.5b)**:**
- Supine on a pillow to start.
- Roll the patient away from the therapist.
- Patient's elbows are folded over each other.

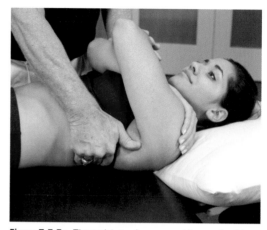
Figure 7.5.5a: Therapist reaches around the underside of the patient and contacts the lateral ribs with a lumbrical grip with the non-thrusting hand.

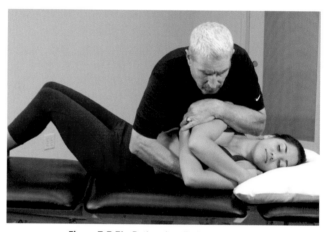
Figure 7.5.5b: Patient is rolled away from the therapist and onto their hand.

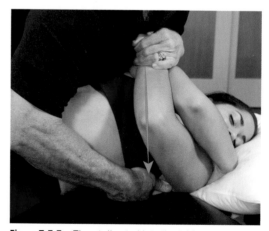
Figure 7.5.5c: Thrust directed into the table toward the therapist's lower hand.

Therapist position (Figure 7.5.5b)**:**
- Standing facing the table next to the patient.

Contact points (Figure 7.5.5a)**:**
- Therapist reaches around the underside of the patient and contacts the lateral ribs with a lumbrical grip with the non-thrusting hand.

- The thrusting forearm will make contact on the lateral side of the folded forearms and upper trunk.

Position for the thrust:
- The patient is rolled away from the therapist and onto their hand.

- Pre-thrust tension will be taken up through the patient's folded arms toward the table. Most of the pre-thrust tension is taken up here.

- The lower hand will increase tension on the ribs by increasing the lumbrical grip tension as a counterforce.

Application of the thrust (Figure 7.5.5c)**:**
- The thrust will be directed into the table toward the therapist's lower hand.

Fine-tuning and keys to success:
- The patient should be right at the edge of the table so when they are rolled away the therapist is not forced to reach over farther than necessary.

- The therapist will need to stand facing across the table with the foot on the thrusting side back. This will give the therapist the greatest stability when performing this technique.

- Success of this technique relies heavily upon the therapist's ability to apply a firm lumbrical grip to the patient's lateral ribs.

- The therapist will superimpose his body over the thrusting forearm for greater control.

- Increasing your grip on the lateral ribs as well as tightening down the thoracic spine from the top through the arms puts you in the best position to effectively perform this technique.

- Make sure the patient is completely rolled onto the lower hand.

- The thrust has to be under control. Speed and low force are essential.

- **Caution:** Most essential is the application of a small amplitude and force to avoid injury to your patient.

- This is a straight translatory movement. Hence, it has to be applied directly into the table.

7.5.6: Seated Mid Thoracic Thrust

Description: The patient is seated at the edge of the table with their arms folded over each other. The therapist stands behind the patient and reaches around with both hands and compresses the thorax both anterior-posteriorly and laterally with your hands and forearms. The therapist leans backward then flexes and/or extends to the affected segment in order to localize the barrier. Additional levers of side-bending and rotation to further engage the barrier are applied. The thrust is applied primarily with tractioning by the therapist through the patient's arms and chest in posterior and superior direction.

When to use: An alternate technique used to restore unilateral or bilateral facet motion in the thoracic spine.

Primary muscle activated: Shoulder extensors and elevators with some trunk rotation to one side.

Suggested tests prior to thrust:
- Palpation for pain and position.
- Seated inspiration and expiration for pain provocation.
- Spring testing.
- Johnston Tap Test.
- PPIVMS/PAIVMs.

Patient position (Figure 7.5.6a)**:**
- Patient is seated at the edge of table close to therapist. Patient's arms are folded over each other with the elbows together.

- The patient should be as close to the table edge as possible so as to allow the therapist easy access. You should not have to reach across the table to hold the patient.

Therapist position (Figure 7.5.6a)**:**
- The therapist stands at table behind the patient with one leg back.

Contact points:
- The therapist's chest contacts affected segment with their pectoral area unilaterally.

- The therapist's arms wrap around the patient with hands around their elbows. Simultaneously, the therapist's forearms contact the patient's lateral thorax below their shoulders.

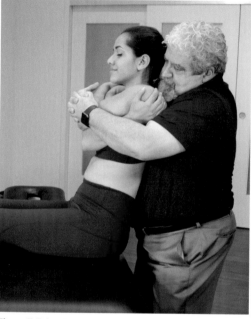

Figure 7.5.6a: Patient seated with arms folded and elbows together, and therapist contacts thorax with chest and wraps arms around patient.

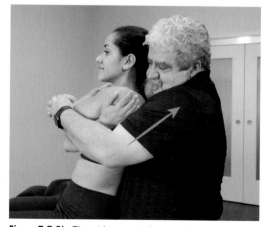

Figure 7.5.6b: Thrust in a posterior-superior direction.

Position for thrust:

- The patient's thoracic spine is flexed to locate the segment. This is felt through the therapist's chest. A towel can also be used to fix this point.

- Additional compression is added through the patient's arms and through contact of lateral thorax by the therapist's arms.

- The therapist's arms should be staggered so as to be able to apply focused lateral translation/compression.

- The therapist pulls the patient back toward them, extending the patient's thoracic spine.

- The patient's thorax can be side-bent away and rotated to the same side you are treating to further engage the barrier.

Application of the thrust (Figure 7.5.6b):

- Gathering pre-thrust tension through the patient's arms and chest, the thrust is applied in a posterior-superior direction.

- Simultaneously, the therapist rotates their chest into the side of the patient's thorax that is rotated toward them.

Fine-tuning and keys to success:

- The table height should be adjusted so that the seated patient's shoulders will be at a level of the therapist's axillae. This will allow the therapist to be in the best position to effectively apply the thrust without having to reach too far over.

- Placing the therapist's foot back provides maximum support, leverage, and control prior to positioning for thrust.

- A small rolled towel can be substituted for chest contact for females and for those not comfortable using chest contact.

- The therapist will flex and extend the thoracic spine in order to effectively locate the affected segment.

- With larger individuals, gripping around their single elbow is an acceptable alternative.

- Lateral compression by the therapist's staggered forearms into each side of patient's lateral thorax is used to provide a translatory compression for additional "focusing."

- Remember that direction and amplitude is critical. Avoid lifting the patient off of the table when applying the traction portion of the thrust.

- It is permissible to let the patient fully exhale and hold prior to the thrust. Speed and the effective use of your body to provide the counterforce and the thrust is absolutely essential for the success of this technique.

7.6: Ribs

7.6.1: Supine First Rib Thrust

Description: The patient is supine with the therapist standing at the head of the table. The therapist turns the patient's head to one side, allowing for placement of the MCP of the index finger of the thrusting hand to contact the first rib. By taking up the slack through the tissue over the rib it causes the head to come back into neutral. Ipsilateral side-bending and contralateral rotation of the neck is introduced. The thrust is applied in an anterior, medial and caudal direction while the therapist's opposite hand applies vertex compression to the skull to reach the barrier. It is more difficult to do but probably avoids some of the pitfalls of positioning and moving the head and neck in space.

When to use: This technique is applied to move a first rib that is elevated or not moving.

Primary muscles activated: Shoulder flexors of thrusting arm. Shoulder flexors of non-thrusting arm.

Suggested tests prior to thrust:
- Palpation for pain and position.
- Palpation during respiration.
- Spring testing for motion.

Patient position (Figure 7.6.1a):
- Patient is supine on table with head on a pillow.

Therapist position (Figure 7.6.1a):
- Therapist stands at the head of the table with one leg back.

Contact points:
- Second MCP of thrusting hand makes contact with the superior aspect of the first rib.

- The opposite hand makes contact with the vertex of the patient's head.

Position for the thrust:
- After contact by the second MCP is made on the first rib, ipsilateral side flexion followed by contralateral rotation of the neck is made until the barrier is engaged.

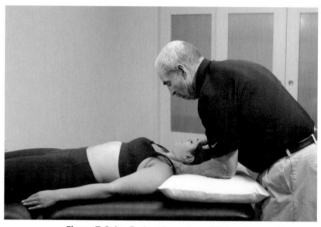

Figure 7.6.1a: Patient is supine with head on a pillow and the therapist stands at the head of the table and slightly toward the side to be treated.

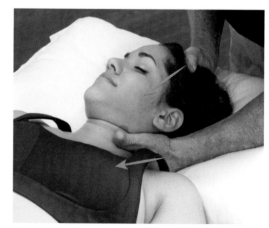

Figure 7.6.1b: Thrust is applied through the first rib in an anterior, inferior and medial direction toward the patient's opposite hip. Compression in the vertex with the opposite hand is applied simultaneously.

Application of the thrust (Figure 7.6.1b)**:**

- The thrust is applied through the first rib in an anterior, inferior and medial direction toward the patient's opposite hip.

- Compression in the vertex of the patient's head with the opposite hand is applied simultaneously with the thrust producing both compression and ipsilateral side flexion to the patient's neck to further engage the barrier.

Fine-tuning and keys to success:

- Patient should lie so that their head is as close to the edge of the table head as possible. This will allow the therapist to be as close to the patient as possible to more easily access the contact areas.

- Table should be at a height that is at least above mid-thigh level. This will put you at the best position biomechanically to perform the thrust.

- Prior to making contact with the first rib it is suggested that you turn the patient's head to the contralateral side to allow better access to the patient's first rib.

- Gathering the tissues over the first rib (mostly the upper traps), your hand will be directed into the table. This will cause the head to move back into the midline as you make contact with the rib through these tissues.

- The head can be moved into the pillow to protect the C spine. This produces retraction of the cervical spine and will serve to protect it from going into too much unwanted extension.

- It is important to line the forearm of the thrusting hand in the direction of the thrusting hand to have the best success.

- This is a two-hand technique. Greater success is guaranteed when both hands work simultaneously.

- The compression with the therapist's vertex contact hand needs to be under control and needs to only apply enough force to engage the barrier but not so much to produce excessive side-bending in the neck.

7.6.2: Supine Second Rib Technique

Description: This is a rather complex technique that requires the simultaneous timing of several movements to accomplish. The patient is placed supine with their arms folded low on their chest. The therapist's thrusting hand is placed so that its ulnar border rests along the anterior second rib with the fingers resting on the patient's anterior shoulder. The therapist contacts the second rib from below with the thenar eminence of their bottom hand. The therapist uses the patient's arms to leverage through the trunk as they apply the thrust. With their thrusting hand, the therapist simultaneously applies a force both to the patient's second rib and shoulder, while their bottom hand and forearm pronate as the patient lifts their head off of the pillow.

When to use: This is used primarily to free up a stuck second rib from the posterior. This technique has less success with heavier persons and those with excessive upper thoracic kyphosis.

Primary muscles activated: Trunk through abdomen, pectorals of thrusting arm. Forearm pronators of lower hand.

Suggested tests prior to thrust:
- Spring test for motion.
- Palpation for position and pain.
- Johnston Tap Test to rule out facet involvement.
- Palpate rib during respiration for movement.

Patient position (Figure 7.6.2a):
- Patient is supine on table with their head on a pillow.

- The patient is moved toward edge of table nearer to the therapist.

- The patient's arms are folded across their chest with forearms together, low across their chest.

- The far arm is usually placed on top.

Therapist position (Figure 7.6.2a):
- Standing at the side of table opposite to side of the rib to be treated.

Contact points:
- The meaty part of the thenar eminence of the therapist's non-thrusting hand is placed over the angle of the of the patient's second rib.

- The therapist's thrusting hand is placed with their hypothenar resting along the anterior second rib with fingers wrapping around the patient's anterior shoulder.

- The therapist contacts the patient's folded arms with their upper abdominal area.

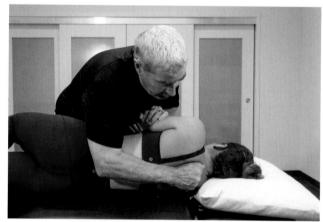

Figure 7.6.2a: Patient is supine with head on a pillow and the therapist applies the meaty part of the thenar eminence over the angle of the patient's second rib.

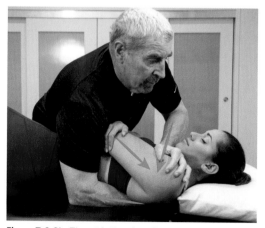

Figure 7.6.2b: Thrust is timed so that, as the lower hand pronates under the rib, the patient's head lifts off the table. Thrust is directed in a superior direction toward the patient's opposite shoulder.

Position for thrust:

- The therapist tightens up at the contact points by adding tension through both of their hands and their trunk.

- The patient's head should be held in the sagittal plane prior to lifting it from the pillow, but it can also be turned toward the side of rib being treated if necessary.

- The therapist's bottom hand will apply traction caudally to the second rib prior to and during the thrust.

Application of the thrust (Figure 7.6.2b)**:**

- The therapist times the thrust so that, as the lower hand pronates under the rib, the patient's head lifts off the table. The thrust is made simultaneously with the therapist's top hand and trunk directing a force in a superior direction toward the patient's opposite shoulder.

- The thrust is accomplished with 80 percent use of the therapist's body, 15 percent with their lower hand and five percent with their upper or thrusting hand.

Fine-tuning and keys to success:

- It is helpful to place the patient four to six inches or a fist width from the edge of the table for consistent positioning for each treatment.

- You do not want the patient too close so as to put yourself at a disadvantage biomechanically and to have the patient fearful of rolling off of the table toward you.

- The therapist should stand to the side of the table near the patient's thorax facing diagonally toward the patient's opposite shoulder so as to be in line with the direction of the thrust.

- The table should be at a level equal to the bend in the therapist's hips.

- The leg on the side of the thrusting hand should be back.

- The contact points here are critical for success. The top hand has to be along the rib but at the same time the hand itself has to have a wide grip over the patient's anterior shoulder on the treatment side.

- Avoid applying the pressure over the clavicle directly. This can be a very sensitive and painful area.

- The bottom hand is on the angle of the rib and has to be medial to the scapula.

- The thenar eminence of that hand has to be made more full to ensure better contact with great comfort to the patient.

- Gathering tension is accomplished with three things occurring simultaneously: the lower hand pronates, the therapist's trunk moves into the folded arms of the patient with their trunk, and pressure is applied with the therapist's thrusting hand that is resting over the anterior second rib and shoulder. The thrust timing is critical with simultaneous movement of all three of these contact points.

- Make sure the thrust is through the rib and not the clavicle or anterior humeral region of the shoulder.

- Do not bend through the hips when applying the thrust. You lose power and control.

- Stay as upright as possible. Keeping the head as upright as possible will help you with maintaining an erect posture, control, and maintenance of your core during the thrust.

- It is essential that you perform the thrust just as the patient starts to lift their head off of the table. You also can time this with breathing.

7.6.3: Supine Mid Rib Thrust

Description: The patient is supine with arms folded over each other. The therapist contacts the affected rib angle and performs a skin lock with their thenar eminence of the non-thrusting hand. The therapist's thrusting forearm contacts the patient's forearms. The patient's thorax is flexed up to the affected rib. The therapist takes up the slack to engage the barrier and applies a thrust along the long axis of the rib in a direction across the patient's body toward their opposite shoulder. This is very similar to the position of performing a thoracic thrust to the facets except the bottom hand is out on the angle of the rib.

When to use: This is used to treat rotated ribs. This will be evident when palpating the angle. It will be more prominent due to rotation than the adjacent ribs. This technique is used to target the third through sixth or seventh ribs. It is a gapping technique of the ribs targeting the costovertebral and costotransverse joints.

Primary muscles activated: Trunk and shoulder protractors on thrusting arm and the shoulder abductors of the opposite hand.

Suggested tests prior to thrust:
- Palpation for position and pain.
- Springing for motion.
- Rotexion/latexion tests for assessing pain and loss of motion.
- Johnston Tap Test to rule out facet involvement.
- Palpate during respiration.

Patient position (Figure 7.6.3a)**:**
- The patient is supine on table with their head on a pillow with their arms crossed over each elbow.

- Usually the far arm is on top.

Therapist position (Figure 7.6.3a)**:**
- Standing at side of bed next to the patient's thorax facing diagonally toward their opposite shoulder with one leg back.

Contact points:
- The therapist's thenar eminence of bottom (non-thrusting) hand makes contact with the angle of the affected rib.

- The patient's folded forearms are contacted by the therapist's forearm of the top (thrusting) forearm.

Position of the thrust:
- A skin lock is made with your bottom hand over the angle of the rib as you traction it away from you with the same hand.

- Slack is taken up to engage the barrier by pushing the patient's arms with your thrusting forearm to gather tension.

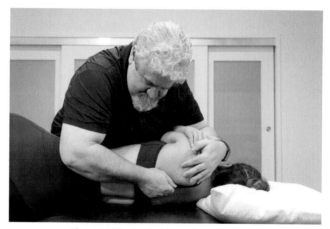

Figure 7.6.3a: Patient is supine with head on a pillow and arms crossed. Therapist applies a skin lock with the bottom hand over the angle of the rib to be treated.

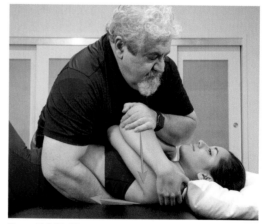

Figure 7.6.3b: Thrust is applied toward and across the table along the long axis of the affected rib toward the opposite axilla, simultaneously applying traction laterally with the lower hand.

Application of the thrust (Figure 7.6.3b)**:**

- Keeping your trunk upright and once you have engaged the barrier, apply the thrust across the table along the long axis of the affected rib toward the opposite axilla.

- Simultaneously with the thrust, the therapist's lower hand tractions the rib laterally.

Fine-tuning and keys to success:

- It is helpful to place the patient four to six inches or a fist width from the edge of the table for consistent positioning for each treatment. This will prevent the patient from having a fear of falling off of the table and will place you in optimal position to provide the treatment.

- It is important to keep your head up and your trunk as upright as possible when getting into position to perform the thrust.

- The leg on your thrusting side is back to provide the best stability in applying the thrust.

- The skin lock is important to fix onto the rib in order to get a good purchase on it.

- It is important to note that the angle of inclination of the ribs changes from the top down. The upper ribs are more horizontal than the lower ones. Hence, when you place your thenar eminence on the rib, its angle of inclination will change as you move down the thorax.

- When rolling the patient toward you we recommend bending their knee on the affected side. This makes it easier to roll the patient toward you with less effort, especially with the larger patient.

- The barrier is best engaged by gathering tension through the patient's forearms with your thrusting forearm and applying tangential tension or force along the long axis of the rib in a lateral direction from the spine.

- Do not lay patient over the hand until the moment of thrust to avoid excessive pressure on the patient's rib cage.

- Keep your head upright to maintain an upright posture.

- It is helpful for the therapist to pinch their shoulder blades together to further stabilize their trunk prior to the thrust.

- Do not thrust by bending through the hips. Power is lost there. It is essential that you use the body to help with the thrust. This gives you more control and requires less effort than using the arms alone.

- The thrust is made toward the opposite side of the table in a more cephalic direction toward the patient's axilla.

- You can also further engage the barrier if needed by adding trunk ipsilateral side-bending, directional eye movements, neck rotation, etc.

- Additionally, adding both patient and therapist breathing may also help to engage the barrier.

7.6.4: Supine Lower Rib Thrust

Description: This supine technique is used to access the lower ribs but not the floating ribs. The patient is supine on the table with their arms folded in front of them. The therapist contacts the affected rib at the angle and applies a skin lock to it with their thenar eminence. The therapist flexes the patient's trunk down to the rib to engage the barrier. This may involve lifting the patient's trunk off of the table. The therapist's thrust is made using their trunk in a direction along the long axis of the affected rib.

When to use: Best used on ribs 7-10 to restore motion. It becomes more difficult the lower you go and is dependent on the size and flexibility of the patient. It is better used on average to smaller individuals rather than large barrel-chested persons. This will involve some lifting of the patient's thorax into flexion off of the table.

Primary muscles activated: Trunk and shoulder depressors of thrusting arm. Shoulder extensors and abductors of opposite arm.

Suggested tests prior to thrust:
- Palpation for pain and position.
- Palpation during respiration.
- Johnston Tap Test to rule out facet involvement.
- Spring testing for mobility.

Patient position (Figure 7.6.4a):
- Supine with their head on a pillow.

Therapist position (Figure 7.6.4a):
- The therapist stands at the side of the table facing toward the patient's opposite shoulder with the leg closest to the table back.

Contact points:
- The therapist's chest/abdomen contacts the patient's folded arms.

- The thenar eminence of your non-thrusting hand will be placed along the angle of the affected rib.

Position for thrust:
- The therapist will reach around the patient's neck and shoulders with the non-thrusting hand and lift the patient into flexion until they reach the rib to be moved.

- The underneath hand will take up additional tension by tractioning along the long axis of the rib.

- You may add side-bending toward you to further gap the rib.

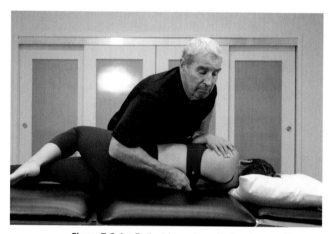

Figure 7.6.4a: Patient is supine with head on a pillow and arms crossed. Therapist applies thenar eminence of lower hand along the angle of the affected rib.

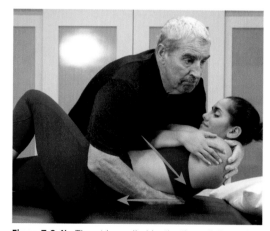

Figure 7.6.4b: Thrust is applied by the therapist's trunk down and away, along the long axis of the affected rib.

Application of the thrust (Figure 7.6.4b):
- Gathering tension through the contact points, the thrust is accomplished by directing it with your trunk down and away from you along the long axis of the affected rib.

Fine-tuning and keys to success:
- It is helpful to place the patient four to six inches or a fist width from the edge of the table for consistent positioning for each treatment. Avoid having them too close as many have a sense or fear they will fall off of the table when you pull them toward you.

- The table should be at a height so that you can bend over it but not so low as to place you in a position where you will have poor mechanical advantage. It should be no lower than your trochanters when you are standing erect.

- Contact points are important. You will be applying the thrust through the patient's arms into your hand. Most of the force will be directed through contact by your chest.

- Prior to thrusting you can side flex the patient toward you to get better a purchase on the rib prior to the application of the thrust.

- Once you are in position to apply the thrust, take up the slack by compression with your chest and tangential pressure with your lower hand.

- The thrust will be performed simultaneously by tractioning with the lower hand away from the spine along the long axis of the affected rib.

- Make sure you do not position the patient over the contact hand until just before applying the thrust. This area can be very uncomfortable to the patient if you hold them over their ribs too long.

7.6.5: Seated First Rib Thrust

Description: The patient is seated on a low table with the therapist behind them. The therapist places one foot on the table and drapes the patient's contralateral arm and shoulder over their knee. The patient naturally leans over the therapist's knee producing some ipsilateral side-bending at the CT junction area. The therapist places their non-thrusting hand on the patient's frontal-parietal region of their head. The same forearm rests in contact with the side of the patient's head, anterior enough so the same elbow sits to the front of the patient's clavicle. With that hand, retract the neck to protect the cervical spine while the other hand contacts the top of the affected rib with the therapist's metacarpal-phalangeal (MCP) of their index finger. The therapist applies a thrust in an inferior, medial and anterior direction using their metacarpal-phalangeal (MCP) of the index finger. Simultaneous counterforce is applied with the non-thrusting hand by compression through the skull. This technique allows the therapist to have good control of all of the levers while protecting the cervical spine.

When to use: This is a good technique for restoring motion to a superior fixed rib dysfunction.

Primary muscles activated: Pectorals, elbow extensors and shoulder protractors of thrusting arm. Shoulder extensors of non-thrusting arm.

Suggested tests:
- Palpation of position of rib.
- Inspiration with palpation.
- Active motion testing of CT area.
- Spring test for motion.

Patient position (Figure 7.6.5a):
- Seated on table's edge with table or stool at a height just above your knees.

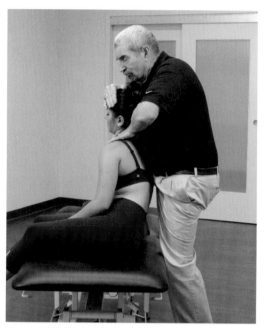

Figure 7.6.5a: Patient is seated on table's edge and therapist stands behind the patient with one foot up on the table.

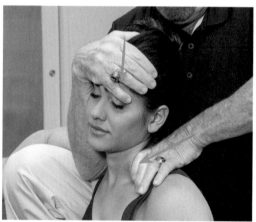

Figure 7.6.5b: Thrust is applied onto the superior surface of the first rib in an inferior, anterior and medial direction.

Therapist position (Figure 7.6.5a):
- Standing behind the patient slightly to the side that will be thrust.

Contact points:
- Second MCP of thrusting hand makes contact over the affected first rib.

- The other arm with bent elbow is draped over the patient's opposite shoulder and clavicle, while the hand rests over the frontal-parietal region of the patient's skull with forearm resting on the side of the patient's face.

Position for the thrust:
- The patient is side-bent ipsilaterally to the CT region. The C spine is rotated contralaterally to the barrier.

- The patient's head is retracted, eliminating the lordosis in the neck.

- Ask the patient to drop their shoulder. Using expiration primarily you have about three seconds before the shoulder comes back up.

Application of the thrust (Figure 7.6.5b):
- The thrust is applied onto the superior surface of the first rib in an inferior, anterior and medial direction.

- The non-thrusting hand applies compression through the vertex to produce a little controlled side-bending as a counterforce.

Fine-tuning and keys to success:
- Patient should be seated as close to the edge of the table as possible.

- The patient's legs can be folded or in the long sit position with the legs over the side.

- Have the patient sit as erect as possible to reduce CT kyphosis.

- The height of the table is important as this requires that the therapist put his foot up on the table.

- It places the patient in the most efficient biomechanical position to apply treatment.

- It is very important to retract the cervical spine with the non-thrusting hand in order to protect the cervical spine. This opens up the cervical facets and prevents the compression from above from closing them down.

- In order to do this with some success, the placement of the arm with flexed elbow over the clavicular area is a must. This helps you to retract the patient's neck easier. Your axilla will rest over the patient's upper traps. This allows for better control in positioning the neck prior to the thrust.

- Make sure that the thrusting hand is not on the upper traps directly. You must move the muscles out of the way to contact the first rib.

- Compression with the non-thrusting hand is done so that ipsilateral side-bending is introduced as a counterforce to the thrust.

- It is important to control and/or limit too much ipsilateral side-bending as you risk injury to the brachial plexus.

- Keeping the thrusting forearm in line with the direction of the thrust will also help limit too much side flexion.

- The thrust is best performed with the patient performing an expiration once the shoulder has dropped.

Description: This is a seated technique that uses a superiorly directed thrust of the affected rib toward the ceiling in the seated position. It can be complicated when first viewed. The patient sits on the edge of either end of the table with their arms folded in front of them. The therapist hooks the ulnar border of the thrusting hand under the angle of the affected rib. The therapist's other hand reaches over the top of the patient's ipsilateral shoulder and grasps the patient's opposite arm or elbow. Then the therapist pivots his body in the opposite direction where he started allowing the patient to drop their head onto his non-thrusting shoulder. This movement by the therapist causes the patient to move into extension and side-bending on the affected side, allowing the therapist a better purchase on the rib. The thrust is made with the therapist's hypothenar onto the rib directed toward the ceiling.

When to use: This technique is used to move a fixed mid rib. It usually works on the fourth through the ninth ribs. This is probably the limits of each end but will depend how accessible the ribs are. It is not a technique one has great success with on very large people.

Primary muscle activated: Shoulder flexors with the rib lift from thrusting arm.

Suggested tests prior to thrust:
- Johnston Tap Test to rule out facet involvement.
- Palpation for pain and position.
- PPIVMs/PAIVMs.
- Quadrant testing.
- Spring test for motion.

Patient position (Figure 7.6.6a):
- Seated at one end of the table with legs over the side.

- Arms are folded in front of the patient's chest below their breast area.

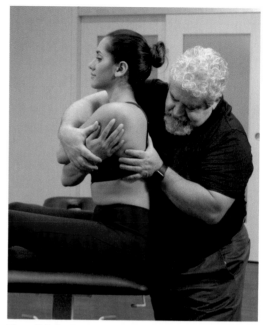

Figure 7.6.6a: Patient is seated at edge of table with arms crossed and therapist stands behind the patient and reaches one arm over the patient's opposite shoulder to grasp arm and hand.

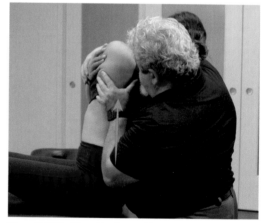

Figure 7.6.6b: Thrust is directed in a superior direction toward the ceiling under the angle of the affected rib.

Therapist position (Figure 7.6.6a):
- Standing in back of patient biased to the side you will thrust.

Contact points:
- The ulnar border of the thrusting hand will contact the underside of the angle of the affected rib.

- The other arm will reach over the top of the patient's contralateral shoulder and grasp the patient's ipsilateral elbow.

Position of the thrust:
- Patient is side-bent and rotated contralaterally so as to expose the affected rib better.

- The therapist will pivot and turn their feet in the opposite direction from where they started to be in position to provide the thrust. This will allow the patient to let their head fall back on the shoulder of the therapist's non-thrusting arm.

- This pivot will allow the patient to go into extension and side-bending of the opposite direction over the therapist's hand.

Application of the thrust (Figure 7.6.6b):
- The thrust is directed in a superior direction toward the ceiling under the angle of the affected rib.

Fine-tuning and keys to success:
- Make sure patient scoots all of the way back to the edge of the table.

- The patient should be at the end of the table that corresponds to the side that will be treated. This allows the therapist easier access to the patient's rib without being impeded by the table.

- The therapist should only raise the table so the patient's iliac crests are not higher than theirs in sitting.

- The positioning of the thrusting hand is critical here. Prepositioning the ulnar border around the rib in such a way that the palm is facing up will ensure success.

- Use your body to initiate the side-bending and rotation away. Pivoting to the side of the thrust with your body allows you to get into a position to apply the thrust. Being able to pivot your body around to get under the rib is essential to positioning for the thrust.

- Having the patient dropping their head over your opposite shoulder is important as it allows the patient to be effortlessly placed into the correct position for the application of the thrust.

- Speed is absolutely critical here. It, along with controlled amplitude taking care not to lift the patient off of the table, will ensure specificity and eliminate moving other parts in the trunk unintentionally.

7.6.7: Seated Anterior Rib Technique

Description: This is a very gentle technique with the patient seated. It uses compression and tractioning to the anterior rib to accomplish the movement. The patient is placed in the seated position back at the edge of the table. The therapist reaches under the patient's axillae and grabs the patient's right thumb in their hand (if you are addressing a right rib) and placing their thenar eminence over the affected rib. The therapist's other hand grabs the patient's opposite thumb and superimposes this hand over the first hand onto the patient's affected rib. Compression is provided both in an anterior and posterior direction with your contact hands and laterally with your forearms to fully engage the barrier. The thrust is applied over the affected rib with compression in posterior superior direction. This technique can also be done standing (Figure 7.6.7d).

When to use: This is a great alternative to use for the upper one or two ribs. Sometimes it works on the third rib. It can be used to treat both an anterior rib and posterior rib dysfunction. By virtue of the compression from both ends of the rib it can effect movement. This is also a good alternative when supine and other seated techniques do not work, or with patients who cannot rest on their back.

Primary muscles activated: Elbow flexors, shoulder extensors and retractors.

Suggested tests prior to thrust:
- Palpation over tender area for pain and movement.
- Johnston Tap Test to rule out facet involvement.
- Springing over ribs.
- Check for rib movement with breathing.

Patient position (Figure 7.6.7a)**:**
- Seated on table. Move patient back on the table toward you.

Therapist position (Figure 7.6.7a)**:**
- Standing behind the patient with one foot back.

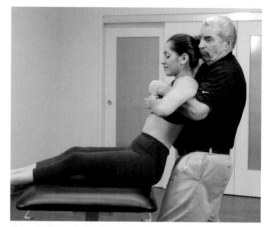

Figure 7.6.7a: Patient is seated on the table and therapist stands behind the patient.

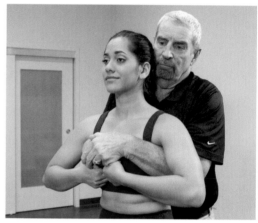

Figure 7.6.7b: Anterior surface of affected rib is contacted by the thenar eminence of the thrusting hand (in this case, right hand).

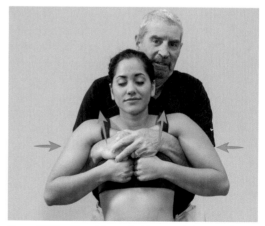

Figure 7.6.7c: Thrust is applied in a posterior superior direction using compression through the therapist's superimposed hands over the patient's affected rib. There is simultaneous compression with the forearms into the patient's lateral ribs.

Contact points (Figure 7.6.7b):
- Anterior surface of affected rib with the thenar eminence of the thrusting hand.

- Therapist's chest.

- The inside of both of the therapist's arms and forearms are wrapped around the patient's thorax anteriorly and laterally.

Position for thrust:
- The therapist reaches around the patient's thorax under the patient's axillae with both hands.

- Grasp the patient's ipsilateral thumb on the treatment side.

- The therapist places their thenar eminence onto the affected rib while holding the patient's thumb.

- The therapist superimposes their opposite hand while grasping the patient's opposite thumb over their thrusting hand.

Application of the thrust (Figure 7.6.7c):
- The thrust is applied in a posterior superior direction using compression through

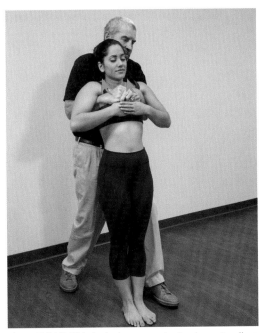

Figure 7.6.7d: This technique can also be done standing.

the therapist's superimposed hands over the patient's affected rib. Simultaneous compression is provided over the lateral ribs during the thrust.

Fine-tuning and keys to success:
- It is important that the table height is such that you get the best biomechanical advantage because there is posterior and some superior movement required of the thrust. The patient's shoulders should just below your axillae.

- Placing one foot back gives you the stability and control to pull the patient up and back toward you.

- You must compress the rib through your hands into you while simultaneously compressing laterally into the patient's thorax. This will help create tension and engage the barrier better prior to the thrust.

- When you reach around the patient, make sure you reach around under the patient's arms. This allows you to apply direct compression to the rib cage and will keep the arms out of the way.

- As you apply the compression anteriorly and laterally with your arms you will lean back toward your hind leg to create pre-thrust tension.

- Holding on to the patient's thumbs gives you better control and allows you to get the patient's arms out of the way with little effort.

- The direction of the thrust up and back in a scooping like motion will be most effective by adding slight supination of the forearms.

- You must make sure that you maintain constant compression both anteriorly and laterally throughout the application of the thrust.

- Normally, if there is audible articulation it will sound like it is coming from the posterior rib attachment.

7.6.8: Prone Lower Rib Thrust

Description: This is a prone technique used to access the lowest ribs. It requires the coordination of lifting the pelvis from below and moving the ribs from above as a counterforce. It is one that you can get in trouble with if too much force is applied because it is directed at your floating ribs. The patient is placed in prone on the table. The treatment involves moving the lower rib on the opposite side away from you. The therapist's thrusting hand ulnar border is placed along the affected lower rib while their opposite hand reaches around and grasps the iliac crest on the same side. The force is applied tangentially along the rib to introduce a gapping or tractioning at the rib attachments. An opposing force is applied on the anterior crest by lifting it away but not off of the table.

When to use: This is used to treat dysfunctions of the eleventh and twelfth ribs.

Primary muscles activated: Shoulder depressors and protractors of the thrusting hand and shoulder elevators and retractors of the non-thrusting hand and trunk rotators.

Suggested tests prior to thrust:
- Palpation for position and pain.
- Spring test for motion.
- Observe breathing.

Patient position (Figure 7.6.8a)**:**
- Patient is prone on the table.

Therapist position (Figure 7.6.8a)**:**
- Therapist stands to the side of the table opposite to the side that will be thrust. The therapist will place the foot back on the side of the thrusting hand.

Contact points:
- Thrusting hand is placed along the long axis of the rib to be treated.

- The other hand will reach around the front of the ASIS on the same side.

Position for the thrust:
- Slack will be taken up to the barrier by pushing into the affected rib along its long axis while lifting the ASIS in a direction away or off of the table.

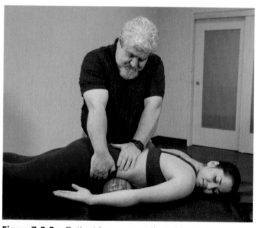

Figure 7.6.8a: Patient is prone on the table and therapist stands to the side of the table opposite to the side that will be thrust.

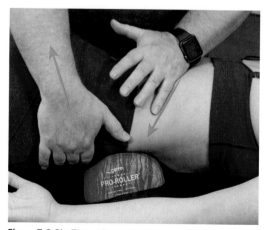

Figure 7.6.8b: Thrust is applied with the left hand away from the therapist along the affected rib, while simultaneously lifting the ASIS to provide counterforce with the right hand.

Application of the thrust (Figure 7.6.8b)**:**
- Once the tension is taken up with both hands on each contact point, a thrust is applied away from you along the affected rib.

- Simultaneous lifting of the ASIS to provide the counterforce will be used.

- The thrust is most controlled and effective by using your body and dropping onto the rib tangentially with your thrusting hand by turning your shoulder toward the rib while the opposite shoulder moves away.

Fine-tuning and keys to success:
- Make sure you move the patient close to your side of the table so it will make it mechanically easier for the therapist to address the rib located on the opposite side.

- You can use a pillow under the patient if there is too much lumbar lordosis when the patient is prone.

- Keeping the foot back on the side of the thrusting hand gives you stability and control.

- The table should be at a height where you can address the rib without bending over when standing erect.

- Keep your head up so as to engage your core.

- It is the lateral border of the hypothenar eminence portion of the hand that makes contact with the angle of the affected rib.

- Be careful not to go too far out on the rib as you will produce too large of a lever and could injure the patient. It is best to make contact just medial to the angle of the rib.

- Get a wide purchase over the ASIS with the other hand. This is a very sensitive area and a good dispersal of forces from the hand will lessen this effect. Cupping the hand over the ASIS is also a helpful way to disperse forces over it and seems to be more comfortable in the author's experience.

- Taking up the slack is easier when you keep your hands on the contact points as extensions of your body and allow your body to produce the movement. You merely turn your upper trunk to build up additional tension. It is critical to use your body to control amplitude and force for success here.

- This is a two-handed technique. The thrust is most successful when the hands move simultaneously, providing counterforce to each other.

- Care must be taken not to push the rib into the table but across the table tangentially, applying a traction force to it. The former can cause a lot of discomfort to your patient.

7.7: Thoracolumbar Junction

7.7.1: Prone TL Junction Traction Thrust in Prone

Description: This is a gentle technique that can be applied to the TL junction using traction with one or two hands. The patient lies prone on their elbows so that their lumbar spine is in slight extension. The therapist contacts the TL junction with a cupped hand, and with the other hand at both ankles. A traction thrust is applied longitudinally in both directions. This can be applied as either a bilateral technique or as a unilateral technique by biasing side-bending in the thorax. This technique may not work as well with a therapist who has a short arm span working on a taller/ longer individual.

When to use: To restore motion at the TL junction.

Suggested tests prior to thrust:
- AROM seated rotation.
- Johnston Tap Test.
- Spring testing.
- Palpation for pain and position.
- PPIVMS/PAIVMs.

Primary muscles activated: Shoulder abductors and depressors bilaterally.

Patient position (Figure 7.7.1a):
- Prone on table.

- The patient will come up and rest on their elbows.

Therapist position (Figure 7.7.1a):
- Standing at the side of the table facing the patient halfway between the patient's ankles and TL junction.

Contact points (Figure 7.7.1b):
- Cupped palm of cephalic placed hand straddles each side of the spinous processes of T12 while the lower hand grasps the posterior ankles.

Position for the thrust:
- The patient will be placed on their elbows while prone.

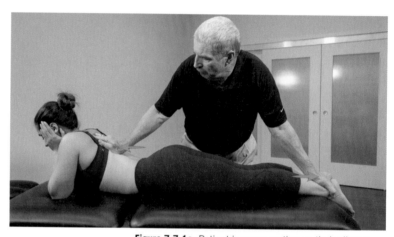

Figure 7.7.1a: Patient is prone resting on their elbows. Therapist places cupped palm of cephalic placed hand straddling each side of the spinous processes of T12 while lower hand grasps posterior ankles. Thrust is applied along the spinous process of T12 into extension with counterforce applied through one or both ankles.

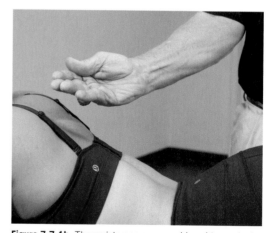

Figure 7.7.1b: Therapist uses a cupped hand to contact the TL junction.

- The patient's feet will be over the edge of the bottom of the table.

- The head will be held up and not flexed.

- Pre-thrust tension will be gathered by longitudinal traction using both hands on the contact areas.

Application of the thrust (Figure 7.7.1a)**:**
- Once the pre-thrust tension is taken up, a small impulse is applied along the spinous process into extension.

- To improve rotation, apply the thrust onto the transverse process.

- Counterforce is applied through one or both ankles with the caudal hand.

Fine-tuning and keys to success:
- The patient's feet need to be off of the table. This reduces any flexion at the knees and allows for a straighter line in the intended direction of the thrust.

- Staggering the placement of the patient's arms can bias them into side-bending to one side or the other.

- The table should be raised so that the patient's buttocks extend no higher than the level of the therapist's iliac crests.

- The therapist will need to bend their trunk to get into the position to apply their hands to the contact points.

- This technique requires that the therapist maintain their core control.

- It is important that the therapist use a cupped hand on the contact point. This allows the spinous process of T12 to rest comfortably within the crease made by the thenar and hypothenar eminences of the hand.

- On some tighter and thinner individuals, the therapist can adjust their hand to a wider base of support for better comfort.

- The therapist can grasp one or both ankles depending on whether they wish to perform a unilateral versus a bilateral technique. The ability to reach the two contact points with taller patients with the hands will be critical for success.

- The best way of taking up the slack with this technique is by leaning forward as you apply traction. The distance between the two hand placements can be significant. Hence, it is better to line up facing the patient's head in order to be in a better mechanical position to apply an effective thrust.

- Once all of the slack is taken up through traction, the thrust is applied by using the shoulders.

- The thrust uses a combination of shoulder abduction and an attempt to lengthen the arms in the direction of thrust and counterforce.

- The generation of enough speed and traction force is critical for success.

- The lower hand has to stay in full pronation if possible.

- It is best to have the patient exhale to relax their muscles.

- Speed is critical for success here.

7.7.2: TL junction Side-lying Rotation Thrust While Stabilizing Entire Lumbar Spine Below

Description: The TL junction is a transitional region where the change in orientation of the planes of the facets can be sudden rather than gradual. Forcing the TL junction into pure rotation can cause unwanted post-treatment discomfort. One way to more effectively manipulate this level is with a side-lying technique that levers the entire lumbar spine as a unit from below. By stabilizing the entire lumbar spine, it serves to protect it by moving it as one unit. It is a combination of rotation with traction technique. The patient is placed in side-lying. The patient's trunk is rotated to the TL junction from above. The therapist's thrusting forearm is placed along the entire lumbar spine to protect it and allow it to move as one when the thrust is made.
The opposite hand moves into the table applying counterforce to the superior segment without compressing the axillary rib cage. Compression by the use of the therapist's body down into the table is performed simultaneously with the thrusting forearm moving toward them and downward to introduce localized movement at the level.

When to use: to restore loss of unilateral rotation in the TL spine.

Primary muscles activated: Shoulder adductors and extensors of thrusting hand. Shoulder depressors and, to a lesser degree, the elbow extensors of the non-thrusting hand.

Suggested tests prior to thrust:
- AROM seated rotation.
- Johnston Tap Test.
- Spring testing.
- Palpation for pain and position.
- PPIVMS/PAIVMs.

Patient position (Figure 7.7.2a):
- Neutral side-lying on table with a pillow under the head.

- The bottom leg is extended while the hip and knee of the top leg are flexed.

- The foot of the top leg is placed behind the knee of the bottom leg.

Therapist position (Figure 7.7.2a):
- Standing facing the patient, lined up closer to the TL junction.

Contact points:
- Top hand and forearm are threaded through the patient's upper most arm and the hand is contacting the upper segment on upper side of the spinous process.

- The forearm of the thrusting (lower) hand is placed along the long axis of the lumbar spine.

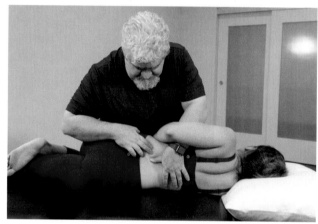

Figure 7.7.2a: Patient is in neutral side-lying with a pillow under the head and therapist takes up axillary hold with left arm and applies body compression onto patient's left hip and pelvis.

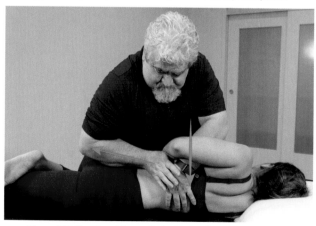

Figure 7.7.2b: Thrust is applied with the forearm along the entire lumbar spine into the table, toward the therapist, and in a caudal direction to achieve slight traction.

Position for the thrust:

- Patient's thorax is rotated away from the therapist down to T12 from the top.

- Then, from below, the segment is rotated to L1 using the forearm of the thrusting hand, and slight traction is applied through a skin lock with the forearm.

- The middle and/or index finger of the thrusting hand will engage the underside of the spinous process on the lamina of L1.

- Further engaging the barrier is accomplished by adding compression through the lower ribs of the therapist onto the patient's thorax.

Application of the thrust (Figure 7.7.2b):

- The thrust is applied with the forearm along the entire lumbar spine into the table, toward the therapist, and in a caudal direction to achieve slight traction.

- The opposite (upper) hand on T12 moves in the opposite direction into the table to provide the counterforce.

- During the application of the thrust, the therapist drops onto the back heel so as to compress the patient's trunk with their lower ribs.

- Add additional compression into the lamina on the underside of the spinous process of L1 with the middle and/or index finger of the thrusting hand.

Fine-tuning and keys to success:

- The patient should always have a pillow under the head to keep the head in neutral so as not to affect the position of segments below.

- The therapist needs to stay upright when performing this thrust as power is lost if the therapist tries to move the patient by bending from their hips.

- Set the table at a height where the top of the therapist's iliac crest is at the same level as the patient's uppermost hip.

- The therapist should keep the foot on the side of their thrusting hand back to gain stability and control.

- The heel of the back foot should be off the ground to accommodate the heel drop.

- The thrusting forearm has to be placed along the entire lumbar spine, as this will be moved as a unit.

- The top hand, with either one or more fingers or the thumb, will be placed on the upper side of the spinous process of T12.

- Slack is taken up with the contact points of the therapist's body as well as the two hands and the forearm of the thrusting hand.

- Compression through resting the therapist's lower ribs on the patient's trunk will further engage the barrier.

- The patient's trunk should be rotated such that it should be perpendicular to the therapist's.

- Do not over rotate the upper thorax during the setup for the technique. It should be sufficient to gently move the scapula closest to the table out of the way so as to clear the table.

- By keeping the head up, the therapist's trunk is maintained in the most erect posture to effectively apply the thrust.

- When the therapist drops onto the back foot during the thrust, it allows best control of the thrust with the body and prevents over rotation.

- This is a technique where you must use your trunk together with your arms. You cannot apply this technique with your arms only, especially with larger patients.

- By rotating the spine as one unit, it ensures that the force is not dissipated through the lumbar spine.

7.7.3: TL Junction Side-lying Rotation Thrust with Gatched Table

Description: This is a side-lying technique that uses the gatched table to add side-bending. The TL junction is localized by gatching the table to localize to the segment. Rotation is provided from the top down to the superior segment. Opposite rotation to the inferior segment is performed from the bottom up. The thrust is applied in pure rotation with the top hand moving into the table while the bottom hand pulls toward the therapist. Compression with the therapist's body toward the table is performed simultaneously with the thrust. The technique is essentially performed in the same direction and method as when the table is flat.

When to use: For loss of unilateral rotation at the TL junction.

Primary muscles activated: Shoulder adductors and extensors of thrusting hand. Shoulder depressors and to a lesser degree the elbow extensors of the non-thrusting hand.

Suggested tests prior to thrust:
- AROM seated rotation.
- Johnston Tap Test.
- Spring testing.
- Palpation for pain and position.
- PPIVMS/PAIVMs.

Patient position (Figure 7.7.3a)**:**
- Side-lying facing the therapist with head on a pillow.

- Table must have a gatched mechanism to raise the patient's head and upper body and provide side-bending at the treatment level.

Therapist position (Figure 7.7.3a)**:**
- Standing next to the table facing the patient.

Contact points:
- Top hand contacts the upper segment on upper side of the spinous process.

- The thrusting hand contacts the segment below on the underside of the spinous process.

- There can be some variations on the hand placement. The ulnar surface of the thrusting hand can also be placed over the lamina on the upper side of the lower segment.

Position for the thrust:
- Begin by placing patient in neutral side-lying.

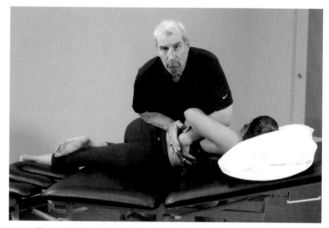

Figure 7.7.3a: Patient is in neutral side-lying with a pillow under the head and table must have a gatched mechanism to raise the patient's head and upper body to provide side-bending at the treatment level.

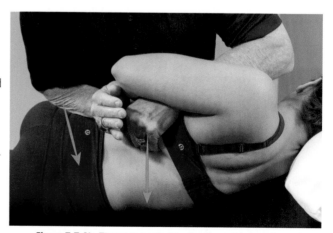

Figure 7.7.3b: Thrust is applied by the therapist dropping onto the back leg and thrusting into the table and toward therapist simultaneously with the thrusting arm.

- Straighten the bottom leg. Flex the top leg at the hip and knee placing the foot behind the knee of the other leg.

- The head of the table is then slowly raised until the segment to be treated is reached, in this case the TL junction.

- The patient's thorax is rotated away from the therapist from the top down to T12.

- Therapist takes up the motion from below by rotating the patient toward them until they reach L1.

Application of the thrust (Figure 7.7.3b)**:**
- The thrust is applied by gathering pre-thrust tension using rotation from below toward the therapist and rotation away from above at the segment.

- At the moment of the thrust, the therapist should drop onto the back leg and thrust into the table and toward them simultaneously with their thrusting arm.

- The upper hand will provide counterforce to the segment above by moving it into the table.

Fine-tuning and keys to success:
- Placing a pillow under the patient's head keeps the head and neck in neutral with the rest of spine. The therapist will position himself closer to the TL junction so as not to create a long lever arm and strain the lumbar spine when they make contact with the spine.

- When the patient is in side-lying, the therapist's iliac crest should line up with the patient's upside hip.

- By placing the thumb on the upper side of the spinous process, the therapist may use a lumbrical grip pushing the fingertips onto the paraspinals nearest the table to guide rotation from above.

- Instead of hooking the underside of the lower segment with the fingers, the therapist can contact the lamina of the transverse process with the ulnar border of the thrusting hand.

- The therapist may further engage the barrier by adding PA pressure into the spine with the thrusting hand.

- Do not over rotate the upper thorax during the setup for the manipulation. The patient's scapula closest to the table should be moved out of the way so as to just clear the table.

- Critical to this technique is that the primary application of compression laterally through the spine must be applied with the therapist's lower ribs.

- This is a two-hand technique. Movement of the hands has to be timed with the drop of the back foot.

- The direction of the thrust has to be into the table and back toward the therapist.

- The patient's trunk should be perpendicular to the therapist's. This places the patient's trunk in the best position to leverage the thrust.

- You cannot effectively perform this technique by using your arms only, especially with larger patients.

- Keep your head up. This helps to maintain an erect posture that is needed to effectively use the body to generate the force needed to perform the thrust.

7.8: Lumbar Spine

7.8.1: Lumbar Rotation in Neutral or Slight Extension

Description: This is what is often referred to as the "lumbar roll." The patient is placed in side-lying facing the therapist. The top leg is bent at the knee and the foot is placed behind the knee of the lower leg. Rotate from the top enough to clear the scapula from the table to the affected segment. Rotate the patient toward you and apply compression through their pelvis with the lower ribs. Once the barrier is engaged, the thrust is accomplished with a combination of compression and rotation with both hands in opposite directions.

When to use: To restore side-bending and rotation on the affected side.

Primary muscles activated: Shoulder extensors and depressors of thrusting arm. Shoulder depressor and pectorals and elbow extensors of opposite arm in combination with a body/trunk drop.

Suggested tests prior to thrust:
- Positional palpation testing.
- PPIVMS, PAIVMs.
- Shear tests as needed.
- Spring testing.
- Quadrant testing.
- AROM.

Patient position (Figure 7.8.1a)**:**
- Side-lying in neutral extension with affected or painful side up.

Therapist position (Figure 7.8.1a)**:**
- Standing facing in a cephalic position along the plane of the intervertebral joints.

- Pre-position with the heel on the thrusting hand side back.

Contact points:
- Top hand at superior segment to be moved on the upside of the transverse process.

- The bottom forearm rests on the upside ilium of the patient.

- The therapist's body below the ribs rests on the patient's pelvis to add compression.

Position for the thrust:
- Extend the patient's bottom leg while flexing the top knee and hip.

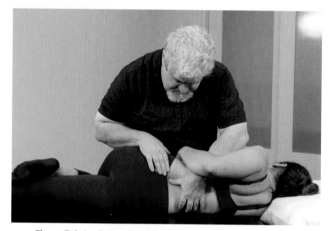

Figure 7.8.1a: Patient is side-lying in neutral extension with affected or painful side up, and therapist takes up axillary hold with left arm and applies body and right elbow compression onto patient's left hip and pelvis.

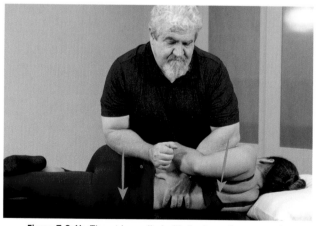

Figure 7.8.1b: Thrust is applied with the lower forearm and lower ribs into the table and down toward the therapist while simultaneously dropping onto the back heel.

- Place the foot of the top leg behind the bend in the knee.

- From the top, move the lower scapula out of the way by rotating the patient's upper trunk away.

- Use the upper hand to rotate down to the targeted segment but not through it.

- From the bottom, rotate the patient in the opposite direction to get to the targeted segment but not through it.

Application of the thrust (Figure 7.8.1b)**:**
- The thrust is applied with the lower forearm and lower ribs into the table and down toward the therapist while simultaneously dropping on to the back heel.

- The therapist adds compression as they drop their body through their ribs onto the patient, aiding rotation.

- A counterforce at the same time is provided with the upper hand applying force into the table with some compression into the lamina of the transverse process on the "up" side of the patient.

Fine-tuning and keys to success:
- Patient should be in neutral side-lying position.

- It is important to allow the patient's upper knee to be a little off of the table so it does not block movement.

- Table height should be such that the therapist's iliac crests are at the same level as the patient's pelvis in side-lying.

- **NOTE:** to get consistent distance between yourself and the patient, use the width of your fist from the edge of the table to the patient's abdomen. For smaller individuals and women, a width of 1.5 to two fists can be used.

- Therapist needs to stand as erect as possible when in contact with the patient to maintain their core.

- The use of an upright posture helps to activate your core.

- The heel of the back foot needs to be off the floor and slightly internally rotated.

- When the thrust is performed, the therapist easily drops the heel and externally rotates the heel and leg back to the neutral position.

- Avoid resting or applying force with the upper arm through the patient's ribs. This can be very uncomfortable.

- Make contact with the pelvis with the softer volar surface of the forearm gathering up tissue to reduce pressure there. Take up the tissue slack with your forearm by pulling the tissue up toward the patient's iliac crest.

- The therapist should rotate the patient's pelvis to around 45 degrees or at least perpendicular to the therapist's trunk. This allows the therapist to be in the most efficient position to perform the thrust from above. They will direct the thrust into the table.

7.8.2: Lumbar Rotation in Flexion with Towel

Description: This side-lying lumbar rotation technique with the spine in flexion is aided by the insertion of a towel to introduce a concave curve on the patient's "down" side on the table. This results in opening up the lumbar facets on the "up" side. The level is located by rotating the patient up to the level while counter-rotating from the top down to the level. Additional flexion is introduced from the top by pulling the patient's "down" arm caudally toward you. This produces additional side-bending into the table. The lower half of the trunk is biased in more flexion by pulling the legs closer or slightly off of the table. The thrust is accomplished using a combination of compression and rotation into the table and is applied with both hands in opposite directions.

When to use: This can be used to open up the facets unilaterally. It can be used in stenosis and some conditions where extension is uncomfortable.

Primary muscles activated: Shoulder extensors and depressors of thrusting arm. Shoulder depressor and pectorals and elbow extensors of opposite arm in combination with a body/trunk drop.

Suggested tests prior to thrust:
- Positional palpation testing.
- PPIVMS, PAIVMs.
- Shear tests as needed.
- Spring testing.
- Quadrant testing.
- AROM.

Patient position (Figure 7.8.2a):
- Side-lying in lumbar flexion.

Therapist position (Figure 7.8.2a):
- Standing facing in a cephalic position along the plane of the intervertebral joints.

- Pre-position with the heel of the thrusting hand side back.

Contact points:
- Top hand at superior segment to be moved on the upside of the transverse process.

- The bottom forearm rests on the upside ilium of the patient.

- The therapist's body below the ribs rests on the patient's pelvis to add compression.

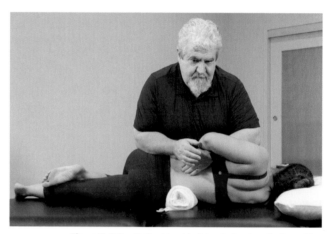

Figure 7.8.2a: Patient is side-lying in lumbar flexion with a rolled towel under the lumbar spine to introduce right side-bending, and therapist takes up axillary hold with left arm and applies body and right elbow compression onto patient's left hip and pelvis.

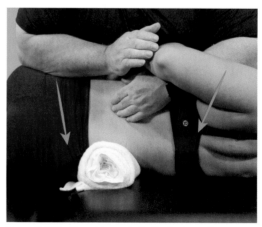

Figure 7.8.2b: Thrust is applied with the lower forearm and lower ribs into the table and down toward the therapist while simultaneously dropping onto the back heel.

Position for the thrust:

- Patient should have their lumbar spine in slight flexion, with no lordosis evident.

- Extend the patient's bottom leg while flexing the top knee and hip.

- Place the foot of the top leg behind the bend in the knee.

- From the top, move the lower scapula out of the way by rotating the upper trunk away.

- Use the upper hand to rotate down to the targeted segment but not through it.

- From the bottom, rotate the patient in the opposite direction to get to the targeted segment but not through it.

Application of the thrust (Figure 7.8.2b):

- The thrust is applied with the lower forearm into the table and down toward the therapist while simultaneously dropping onto the back heel.

- The therapist adds compression as they drop the body through his ribs onto the patient aiding rotation.

- A counterforce at the same time is provided with the upper hand applying force into the table with some compression into the lamina of the transverse process on the "up" side of the patient.

Fine-tuning and keys to success:

- Patient should be in lumbar flexion.

- It is important to allow the patient's upper knee to be a little off of the table so it does not block movement.

- Table height should be such that the therapist's iliac crests are at the same level as the patient's pelvis in side-lying.

- **NOTE:** to get consistent distance between yourself and the patient, use the width of your fist from the edge of the table to the patient's abdomen. For smaller individuals and women, a width of 1.5 to two fists can be used.

- Therapist needs to stand as erect as possible when in contact with the patient to maintain core.

- The heel of the back foot needs to be off the floor and slightly internally rotated.

- When the thrust is performed, the therapist easily drops the heel and externally rotates the heel and leg back to the neutral position.

- Avoid resting or applying force with the upper arm through the patient's ribs. This can be very uncomfortable.

- Make contact with the pelvis with the softer volar surface of the forearm gathering up tissue to reduce pressure there. Take up the tissue slack with your forearm by pulling the tissue up toward the patient's iliac crest.

- The therapist should rotate the patient's pelvis to around 45 degrees or at least perpendicular to the therapist's trunk. This allows the therapist to be in the most efficient position to perform the thrust from above. The therapist will be able to direct the thrust into the table.

- Compression of the lower ribs onto the pelvis of the patient is important for both control and focusing.

- This compression onto the patient has to be simultaneous with the foot drop and the forearm thrust.

7.8.3: Lateral Flexion Thrust Lumbar Spine

Description: This is a side-lying technique that attempts to open the lumbar facet(s) unilaterally by a pure side-bending thrust. The patient is placed in side-lying. Their bottom leg is straightened while the top leg is flexed, allowing the therapist to flex the spine to the affected level. From the top down the trunk is rotated down to the level. The thrust is applied with both hands placed on the "downside" of the transverse processes above and below the affected level to create a fulcrum that produces contralateral lateral flexion there. This side-lying technique requires lots of leverage through the hands to 'open up' the restricted side.

When to use: To restore unilateral side-bending of the lumbar spine.

Primary muscles activated:
Shoulder extensors and depressors of thrusting hand. Pectorals, shoulder flexors, and elbow extensors of non-thrusting hand.

Suggested tests prior to thrust:
- PPIVMS/PAIVMs.
- Spring test.
- AROM.
- Quadrant testing.
- Palpation for pain and position.

Patient position (Figure 7.8.3a):
- Side-lying in neutral with their head resting on a pillow.

Therapist position (Figure 7.8.3a):
- Standing facing the patient with one leg back.

Contact points:
- Top hand contacts the upper segment on the underside of its spinous process.

- The lower hand contacts the lower segment on the underside of its spinous process.

- The therapist contacts the patient's trunk and pelvis with the lower ribs.

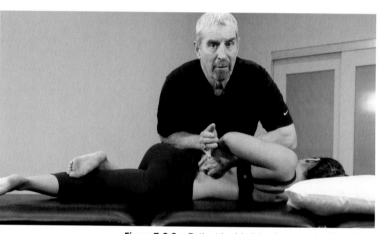

Figure 7.8.3a: Patient is side-lying in neutral with their head resting on a pillow and therapist contacts patient's trunk and pelvis with the lower ribs.

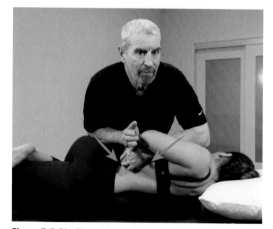

Figure 7.8.3b: Thrust is applied by rapid contralateral lateral flexion through the contact hands simultaneously at the segment while compressing the patient's pelvis with the lower ribs toward each other and into the table.

Position for the thrust:

- The patient's bottom leg is flexed at the hip, placing the bottom foot off of the table.

- The top leg is flexed at the knee and hip with the foot placed behind the knee of the bottom leg.

- Additional flexion is introduced by pulling the patient's bottom arm in a caudal direction.

- The patient is rotated from below to the segment and counter-rotated to the segment from above.

- Local contralateral lateral flexion at the segment is introduced with both hands to open the treatment side.

- Compression is added through the therapist's lower ribs onto the patient's pelvis to take up pre-thrust tension.

Application of the thrust (Figure 7.8.3b):

- The thrust is applied by a rapid contralateral lateral flexion through the contact hands simultaneously at the segment.

- The therapist, while compressing the patient's pelvis with the lower ribs, drops onto the back heel. Simultaneously, they apply pressure with the primary thrusting forearm and hand into the table and toward them.

Fine-tuning and keys to success

- The patient should be placed approximately four to six inches or the width of a fist from the table edge. This ensures a consistent patient position each time you perform this technique.

- The patient's spine needs to be resting in neutral before additional motion is introduced

- The table height should be adjusted for therapist comfort.

- The therapist must maintain an erect posture to make the best use of their core. This is done by keeping the head up.

- The best contact on the spine is to hook the fingers around the underside of superior and inferior segments or over the tissues above the same segment to get leverage. It is as if you are trying to bow or bend at the segment upward.

- The position of the therapist's lower palms acts as a fulcrum to encourage side-bending.

- **Do not try to perform this technique with the hands only.**

- Compression through the patient's pelvis with the lower ribs is essential for this technique. It helps take up pre-thrust tension and provides more efficient leverage for the therapist to perform the technique.

- For larger patients, this will be one of the only ways you can generate any force.

- Timing the compression and the drop simultaneously is essential for success.

7.8.4: Seated Lumbar Traction Thrust

Description: This is a seated technique that requires the therapist to lift the patient from the table and do a quick drop on their heels to apply the thrust. The patient is seated with arms folded low on their chest while at the edge of the table. The therapist reaches around the patient and either entwines their hands around their forearms or beneath them. The therapist stands with one leg back. The patient is flexed to localize to the level. Then the patient is lifted a little off the table and the thrust is accomplished by the therapist dropping straight down on their back foot.

When to use: Use to restore motion in the lumbar spine but also as a traction technique to reduce non-neurological referred pain. This is a traction technique that can be used with the older patient or those with degenerative joint disease that do not respond to rotary techniques. Caution should be used with this technique, as you need to rule out a hypermobility and/or instability below before using this technique as it could exacerbate the problem.

Primary muscles activated: Shoulder elevators and elbow flexors to lift patient. Eccentric contraction of the same with a heel drop to do the thrust.

Suggested tests prior to thrust:
- Springing.
- Palpation for pain and position.
- Quadrant testing.
- AROM testing.
- PPIVMs/PAIVMs.

Patient position (Figure 7.8.4a)**:**
- Seated on table with arms folded over each other.

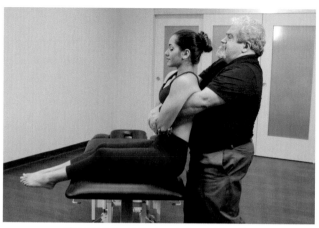

Figure 7.8.4a: Patient seated on table with arms folded over each other and therapist standing behind the patient with one leg back.

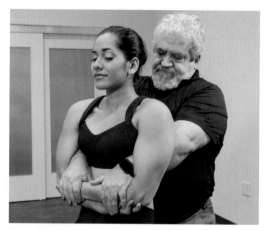

Figure 7.8.4b: Therapist threads hands under the patient's arms to grab both folded forearms.

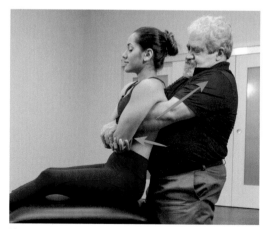

Figure 7.8.4c: Once the patient is lifted, therapist performs a rapid drop onto their back heel to apply the thrust.

Therapist position (Figure 7.8.4a)**:**
- Standing behind the patient with one leg back.

Contact points (Figure 7.8.4b)**:**
- Therapist reaches around and grabs both folded forearms of the patient.

- The therapist's trunk makes contact with the patient's trunk.

Position for thrust:
- Patient is pulled up and back toward the therapist from the table so their buttocks are a few inches off of the table.

- The therapist will lean back and locate the affected segment by flexing the patient to it.

Application of the thrust (Figure 7.8.4c)**:**
- Once the patient is lifted, the therapist drops onto their back heel to apply the thrust.

Fine-tuning and keys to success:
- The patient needs to be as close to the edge of the table as possible so the therapist has access to the patient for the lift.

- The table should be raised so that the patient's shoulders line up just below the axillae of the therapist.

- By placing one foot back, this gives the therapist control to be able to lift the patient using their core.

- The lift is accomplished by wrapping the hands around the patient's arms, or can also be achieved by reaching to the inside of the arms to lift from inside the elbows over the patient's forearms if needed.

- The therapist can use their body to fine-tune the amount of flexion by moving away or toward the table.

- The therapist must be able to get the patient into some extension for this to be successful.

- The thrust has to be directed down and back onto the heel(s).

- The drop has to be quick and as abrupt as possible onto the heel(s). This is done with eccentric contraction of the elbow flexors.

7.8.5: Standing Lumbar Traction Thrust

Description: The patient is standing back-to-back with the therapist. The therapist stands with one foot back with the heels off the floor. The patient folds their arms low on their chest. The therapist backs up to the patient and reaches around to grab the patient's elbows from behind. The therapist bends forward to create a fulcrum for the patient over their back. This will allow the patient's feet to be lifted clear of the floor. The patient is asked to lean their head back and rest it on the therapist's shoulder. A traction force is exerted through the spine by the therapist dropping on to their heels quickly.

When to use: This is good to use for dysfunctions that cause radiating symptoms. It seems to work well on patients that have degenerative changes from aging when regular lumbar rolls do not. Caution should be used with this technique, as you need to rule out a hypermobility and/or instability below before using the technique as it could exacerbate the problem.

Primary muscles activated: Leg muscles simultaneous with a body drop.

Suggested tests prior to thrust:
- AROM.
- Quadrant testing.
- Spring testing.
- Shear testing if needed.
- PPIVMs/PAIVMs.

Patient position (Figure 7.8.5a):
- Standing in an erect posture with their hands folded low on their chest.

Therapist position (Figure 7.8.5a):
- Standing with their back to the patient with one foot back.

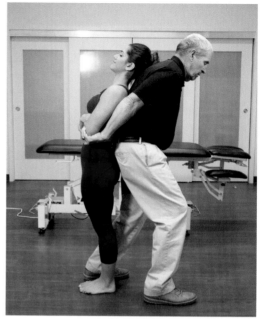

Figure 7.8.5a: Patient standing in an erect posture with their hands folded low on their chest and therapist standing with their back to the patient with one foot back.

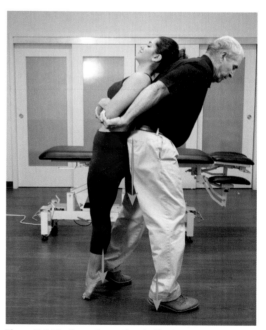

Figure 7.8.5b: Once the patient is lifted, thrust is applied by a quick drop onto the therapist's heels with a body drop.

Contact points:
- Both of the patients elbows are grasped by the therapist.

- The therapist's lower back and buttocks contact the patient's lower back to create a fulcrum with their own back.

Position for the thrust:
- The therapist lifts the patient through the elbows and extends the patient over their back.

- By forward bending, the therapist is able to fulcrum with their own pelvis against the patient's to clear their feet from the floor.

Application of the thrust (Figure 7.8.5b)**:**
- Just before the thrust, the therapist lifts their heels off of the floor.

- The patient is asked to let their head fall back on the therapist's shoulders.

- The thrust is accomplished with a quick drop onto the therapist's heels with a body drop.

Fine-tuning and keys to success:
- Make sure the patient folds their arms across their low chest and not elbow to elbow.

- This allows the therapist to easily reach back and grab the patient's elbow.

- The therapist should not attempt this technique if they are shorter than the patient as getting the proper leverage will be difficult at best.

- This will also not be advised with a heavier person or when both the therapist and patient's morphology will make this technique impossible.

- The best contact point seems to be when the therapist is able to line their own hips/pelvis with the patient to use as the primary fulcrum.

- This may require some stooping on the part of the therapist to line this up correctly.

- For stability sake it is important for the therapist to place one leg behind the other.

- You might have great success by having the patient breathe out just prior to thrusting.

7.8.6: Supine LS Traction Thrust

Description: The patient is placed on their back with the knees bent and their feet flat on the table. The therapist takes their thrusting hand and hooks their fingertips around the base of the sacrum (Figure 7.8.6a) while the other forearm and hand rests over both ASISs. The therapist leans back to take up the slack prior to the thrust. The thrust is performed in a straight caudal direction toward the foot of the table.

When to use: for movement dysfunctions at the lumbosacral spine with the older patient with degenerative changes and those who cannot tolerate rotary or gapping motions.

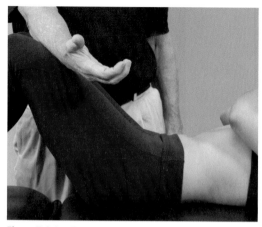

Figure 7.8.6a: Therapist's thrusting hand will hook fingertips around the base of the sacrum.

Primary muscles activated:
Shoulder abductors of thrusting arm and both quads and hip extensors. Shoulder adductors of opposite arm.

Suggested tests prior to thrust:
- PPIVMS, PAIVMs.
- Spring testing.
- Quadrant tests.
- AROM testing.
- Shear testing as needed.

Patient position (Figure 7.8.6b):
- Supine with head on the table.

- The knees are bent with the feet flat on the table.

Therapist position (Figure 7.8.6b):
- Standing at the table near the patient's pelvis.

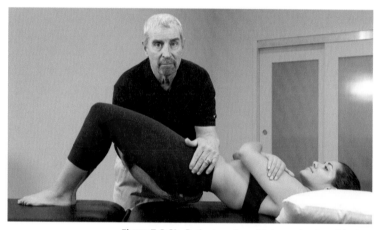

Figure 7.8.6b: Patient supine with knees bent and feet flat on the table. Therapist hooks fingertips around base of the sacrum with the lower hand and contacts patient's ASISs with upper forearm.

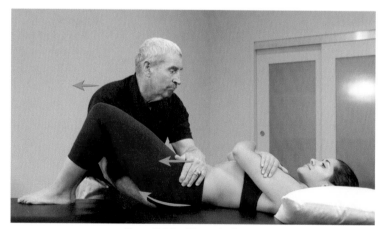

Figure 7.8.6c: Thrust is directed caudally using both hands and the body of the therapist toward the foot of the table.

Contact points:

- Patient's sacrum rests on therapist's palm.

- The therapist's fingertips are hooked over the base of the sacrum.

- The therapist's other forearm and hand rest across the patient's anterior superior iliac spines.

Position for thrust:

- The therapist may have to preposition the patient over the LS junction by having the patient do a bridge and reset their LS area onto the therapist's hand.

- Pre-thrust tension is taken up with the therapist pulling with both hands in a caudal direction.

Application of thrust (Figure 7.8.6c)**:**

- The thrust is directed caudally using both hands and the body of the therapist toward the foot of the table.

Fine-tuning and keys to success:

- Patient positioned with knees bent and their feet flat on the table so this allows them to bridge if needed. It also allows the therapist to reach around or between the patient's knees.

- The therapist should pre-position themselves so their body is facing toward the foot of the table. This will bias them toward the direction of the thrust.

- The therapist must place one leg back to give them the best mechanical advantage when applying a caudal pull into traction.

- The best purchase of the anterior contact points is resting your forearm across the anterior pelvis nestled against the ASIS. This has to be firm.

- The hand will further wrap around the patient's anterior pelvis just above the trochanter to provide better stability.

- It is helpful to have the patient do a pelvic tilt or reverse pelvic tilt to localize the L5-S1 segment over your hand.

- Taking up the slack with the pull on the pelvis and sacral base along with the caudal lean will best set this patient up for the thrust.

- Take up the slack by leaning with the body until the patient's nose moves.

- Two mini thrusts prior to applying the final thrust are helpful to ensuring a better outcome.

- The therapist has to use their body in conjunction with their hands.

- Turning the head in the caudal direction may help facilitate some of this directionality. But it is not necessary.

- You can also turn the toe of the back leg out and the toe of your front leg toward the head of the table to get better stability with the thrust.

7.9: Sacroiliac Joint

7.9.1: Side-lying Posterior Innominate Thrust

Description: The patient is placed in side-lying on the table facing you. Rotate the patient all of the way down to the LS junction so the entire spine is locked to that segment. The therapist places their thrusting hand on the patient's "upside" PSIS while the other hand contacts their lateral shoulder. The thrust is accomplished by the use of the thrusting hand over the PSIS moving down and toward the table. The therapist's body applies compression through the pelvis simultaneously. The non-thrusting hand moves the upper trunk through the shoulder into contralateral side-bending but with no additional rotation.

When to use: To correct a posteriorly fixed innominate.

Major muscles activated: Shoulder depressors/lateral protractors and triceps of upper hand and pectorals and shoulder extensors of thrusting hand.

Suggested tests prior to thrust:
- Fortin's finger test.
- Sacral compression test.
- ASIS distraction test.
- Gaenslen's test.
- FABER's/Patrick's test.
- Thigh thrust/Femoral shear test.

Patient position (Figure 7.9.1a):
- Side-lying on table facing therapist.

Therapist position (Figure 7.9.1a):
- Standing at table facing the patient.

Points of contact:
- Upper hand is on anterior aspect of the upside shoulder.

- The thrusting hand is cupped over the PSIS of the patient's innominate.

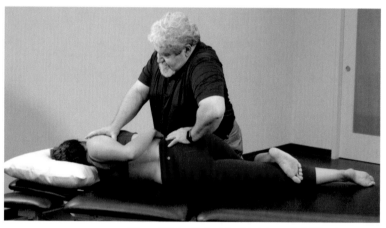

Figure 7.9.1a: Patient in side-lying with full lumbar rotation and therapist facing the patient.

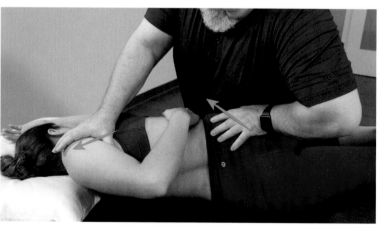

Figure 7.9.1b: The left hand cupped over the patient's PSIS applies the thrust and the therapist uses their body to add compression and force toward the table.

Position for the thrust:

- The patient's lumbar spine is rotated fully from above down to the LS junction.

- Slack is taken up by introducing contralateral side-bending with the non-thrusting hand and anterior rotation of the innominate on the affected side with the thrusting hand to engage the barrier.

Application of the thrust (Figure 7.9.1b)**:**

- The thrusting hand cupped over the patient's PSIS applies the thrust; the therapist uses their body and incorporates compression and force toward the therapist and the table, producing anterior innominate rotation.

- Simultaneously, the upper hand applies counterforce, moving the trunk into contralateral side flexion.

Fine-tuning and keys to success

- Patient should be about four to five inches from the edge of a table or about a width of a man's fist to maintain consistency in positioning your patient.

- The top leg should be slightly off of the table, bent around 60 degrees at the hip.

- The therapist should stand slightly facing cephalically to line up with the long axis of the patient's thigh.

- The thrusting hand needs to be cupped so as to diffuse the pressure over the bony pelvis.

- Be careful with the upper hand contact so that you are not pushing into the chest but rather the shoulder.

- Make sure you have rotated the patient all of the way down into the sacrum because the motion should take place at the innominate.

- The thrust has to use a combination of core and compression with the therapist's body, forcing through the hand simultaneously.

- This, like most of the techniques, is a two-hand technique. The top hand must provide the counterforce to accomplish the technique.

7.9.2: Prone Posterior Innominate Thrust with Leg Off Table

Description: This is a prone technique to treat the innominate that allows for good therapist leverage that will be limited by the table. It is a good technique where a lot of strength is not needed. The patient is placed on the table with one leg hanging over the side with the foot on the floor. The therapist applies a thrusting impulse into the PSIS of the remaining leg simultaneously lifting this leg to provide a counterforce.

When to use: To correct a posterior innominate.

Primary muscles activated: Shoulder depressors of the thrusting side. Shoulder elevators and scapular retractors of opposite side.

Suggested tests prior to thrust:
- Fortin's finger test.
- Sacral compression test.
- ASIS distraction test.
- Gaenslen's test.
- FABER's/Patrick's test.
- Thigh thrust/Femoral shear test.

Patient position (Figure 7.9.2a):
- Prone on table with one leg over the side.

Therapist position (Figure 7.9.2a):
- Standing at the same side of the table facing the patient's mid thorax.

Contact points:
- Thrusting hand is over the PSIS on the side of the leg on the table.

- Opposite hand wraps around the front of the thigh above the knee.

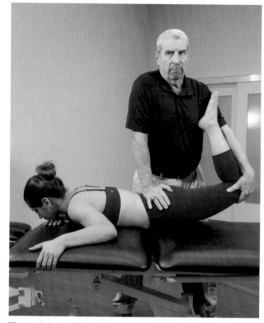

Figure 7.9.2a: Patient is prone on table with unaffected leg over the side. Therapist stands on the same side of the table and places thrusting (right) hand over opposite PSIS and left hand around the front of the thigh above the knee.

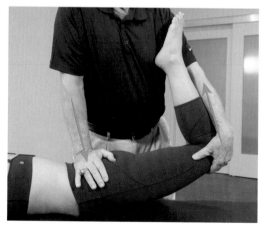

Figure 7.9.2b: Thrust is directed through the patient's PSIS down toward the table.

Position for the thrust:

- Patient's leg that is off the table is flexed at the hip to approximately 90 degrees.

- This will allow the patient's foot to make contact with the ground.

- The other leg is lifted off the table adducting and internally rotating to open up the posterior SI joint to engage the barrier.

Application of the thrust (Figure 7.9.2b):

- The thrust is directed through the patient's PSIS down toward the table.

Fine-tuning and keys to success:

- Patient should be positioned at the table's edge so it allows their leg to easily hang over the table unimpeded.

- Table height: Set at level so that patient's foot that hangs over the side contacts the floor with a slightly bent knee.

- The therapist should stand just behind the patient's "down" leg.

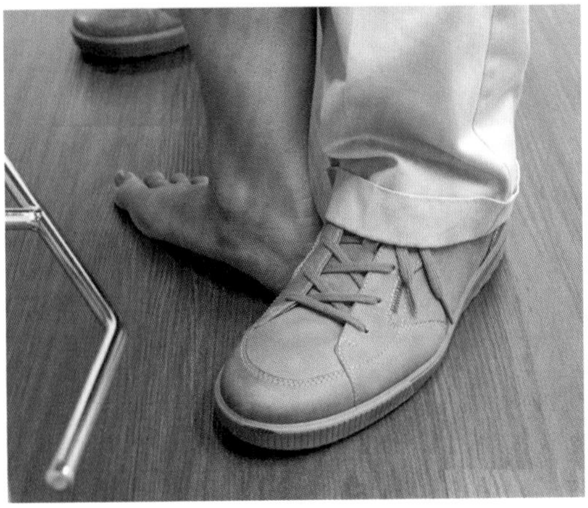

- Therapist's midfoot is placed behind the heel of the patient's, preventing the foot from slipping when the other leg is lifted and the thrust is applied (Figure 7.9.2c).

- A wide handgrip over the PSIS is suggested, as this can be very sensitive to point pressure. A wider dispersal of contact forces will lessen discomfort for the patient.

- In taking up tension, keep the thrusting arm straight.

- You can depress the shoulder of the thrusting hand to add additional tension prior to the thrust.

- Turning the trunk toward the thrusting hand will also help with leverage.

- This is a two-hand technique. Counterforce is applied by lifting the same leg with the non-thrusting hand to maintain tension.

Figure 7.9.2c: Therapist's foot placed behind the heel of the patient's, preventing the foot from slipping when the other leg is lifted and the thrust is applied.

7.9.3: Prone Single-Arm Pushup for Posterior Innominate

Description: This is a technique where the patient is placed prone on the table. The therapist fixes one hand over the PSIS farthest from them and has the patient do a single-arm pushup on that side. A thrust is applied moving the innominate into the table as the patient gathers up tension under the therapist's hand(s) from pushing off the table. Have the patient do two or three single-arm pushups to appreciate tension at the barrier prior to the thrust. The therapist may thrust into the table with one or both hands.

When to use: Effective technique to move a posteriorly fixed innominate. With simultaneous lumbar problems this technique should be used with more caution.

Major muscles activated: Shoulder depressors of thrusting hand(s) depending on whether using one or both hands. A little body drop is also used.

Suggested tests prior to thrust:
- Fortin's finger test.
- Sacral compression test.
- ASIS distraction test.
- Gaenslen's test.
- FABER's/Patrick's test.
- Thigh thrust/Femoral shear test.

Patient position (Figure 7.9.3a):
Prone on table with the far arm primed to do a pushup while the arm closer to the therapist rests on the table.

Therapist position (Figure 7.9.3a):
Standing at the side of the table near the lower thorax facing the patient with one leg back.

Contact points: Thrusting hands over the patient's far PSIS. If using one hand, the opposite hand will be placed on the patient's far shoulder.

Preparation for the thrust: The therapist will ask the patient to perform a single-arm pushup on the side of the dysfunction (far side) while they monitor end feel or tension under their hand or hands. This will depend on whether they are using a one or two hand technique. With the one hand technique, they can guide the single-arm pushup with one hand and assess tension with the thrusting hand.

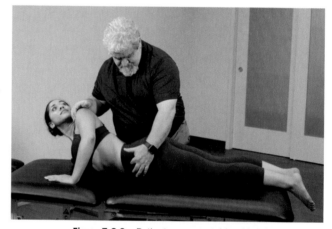

Figure 7.9.3a: Patient prone on table with left arm performing pushup while right shoulder remains on the table.

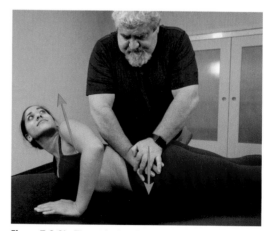

Figure 7.9.3b: Thrust is timed to coincide with patient's pushup and directed down and into the table.

Application of the thrust (Figure 7.9.3b)**:**
- The thrust is applied once tension has been achieved under the thrusting hand(s) down and into the table using a very high velocity, small amplitude impulse.

Fine-tuning and keys to success:
- The patient needs to be as close to the edge of the table and therapist as possible. This will avoid having the therapist bend too far over to engage the contact point on the far ilium. It will serve to avoid compromising body mechanics and mechanical advantage.

- Set the table height so that, when the therapist is standing upright, the finger-tips will touch the table. This will place you in the best mechanical position to apply the correct force and direction.

- The therapist should make sure to contact the patient's PSIS with a cupped palm to disperse forces over that area. This contact point can be quite tender on slender individuals if the forces are not dispersed.

- Have the patient do two to three single-arm pushups on the affected side to build up tension and get a sense of the barrier.

- The therapist can use the non-thrusting hand to help guide this motion while using the thrusting hand to assess tension.

- The thrust is applied by using both the body dropping and the arms that are held in very slight flexion.

7.9.4: Supine Upslip Bent Knee Thigh Pull

Description: This is another SI joint technique where the patient is supine and forces are directed through the thigh. The patient is placed supine with the knee flexed on the affected side. The therapist sits on the patient's foot to stabilize the extremity. One hand is entwined behind the knee while the other is placed on the anterior thigh. The hand behind the knee grasps the forearm of the hand on the thigh. The force is directed through the thigh caudally to avoid stressing the knee joint by the intertwined hand placements on the patient's thigh.

When to use: This is the technique of choice for correcting an innominate upslip when the patient has an issue in the knee or ankle.

Primary muscles activated: Shoulder extensors and to a lesser degree the elbow flexors.

Suggested tests prior to thrust:
- Fortin's finger test.
- Sacral compression test.
- ASIS distraction test.
- Gaenslen's test.
- FABER's/Patrick's test.
- Thigh thrust/Femoral shear test.

Patient position (Figure 7.9.4a):
- Supine on table with knee flexed and the foot flat on the table near the edge.

Therapist position (Figure 7.9.4a):
- Initially standing at the side of the affected SI. Then seated on the patient's distal foot on the treatment side.

Contact points:
- Therapist gently sits over the patient's distal foot on the affected side.

- The therapist's arm closest to the patient is looped behind their knee with their hand making contact with the opposite forearm.

- Then the opposite hand is placed on the patient's affected thigh.

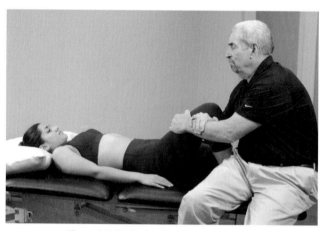

Figure 7.9.4a: Patient is supine with affected knee bent and therapist sits on patient's foot on the treatment side.

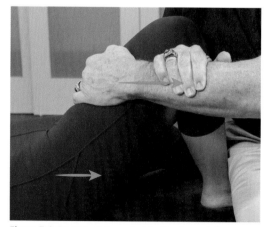

Figure 7.9.4b: Thrust is applied by the therapist's body and arms through the patient's anterior thigh in a caudal direction.

Preparation for the thrust:
- Therapist leans back to take up the slack through the hip and SI joint through the patient's thigh.

Application of the thrust (Figure 7.9.4b):
- A high velocity, low amplitude thrust is made through the patient's anterior thigh in a caudal direction.

Fine tuning and keys to success:
- The patient should rest comfortably with their arms folded and their head on a pillow.

- The therapist should sit on the patient's foot in a way that does not put uncomfortable pressure on it.

- Sitting near the distal end of the patient's foot with either the lower buttocks or upper thigh seems to be most comfortable to the patient and therapist alike.

- By virtue of hand positions, the majority of force is dissipated through both hands so as to avoid doing a drawer test on the knee.

- In order to take up the slack, both leaning back and extension of both shoulders is helpful.

- The thrust should be of such amplitude that, when performed, it only makes the head nod forward.

7.9.5: Leg Pull Thrust for Upslip and Anterior Innominate

Description: This is a general leg traction technique that has been used to treat combinations of one or more sacroiliac dysfunctions and certain lumbar and/or hip dysfunctions. The therapist stands at the foot of the table and takes a hold of the patient's leg near the ankle. The leg is placed in internal rotation and slight adduction as it is lifted off of the table. The force applied is small through the long axis of the leg toward the foot of the table. The patients are able to stabilize themselves by pushing their non-affected foot into the table. For the anterior innominate this thrust can be performed in prone.

When to use: In this case, this technique is used to treat an upslip and anterior innominate.

Primary muscle groups activated: Shoulder extensors and scapular retractors/adductors.

Suggested tests prior to thrust:
- Gaenslen Tests.
- Thigh thrust test.
- ASIS distraction test.
- Sacral compression test.
- Palpation for position.
- Fortin's finger test.

Patient position (Figure 7.9.5a):
- Supine on table with head on pillow.

Therapist position (Figure 7.9.5a):
- Standing at the foot of the table.

Contact point (Figure 7.9.5b):
- Hands wrapped around the patient's ankle above the malleoli.

Position for the thrust:
- Have patient fold arms in front of them.

- Bend the far knee and hip so that the foot is flat on the table.

- Raise the extended leg off of the table about 25 degrees, adduct and internally rotate it at the hip.

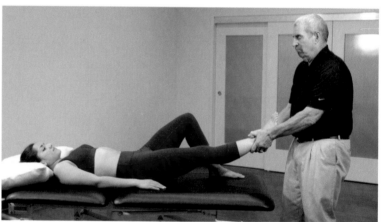

Figure 7.9.5a: Patient is supine with head on pillow and unaffected leg bent with foot flat on table. Therapist wraps hands around the patient's ankle above the malleoli.

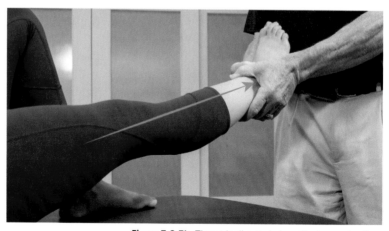

Figure 7.9.5b: Thrust is directed along the long axis of the leg toward the therapist's chest.

Application of the thrust (Figure 7.9.5b)**:**
- The thrust is directed along the long axis of the leg toward the therapist's chest.

Fine-tuning and keys to success
- The patient's leg that remains on the table should be flexed at the knee with the foot flat to allow the patient to push into the table and keep them from sliding down when the thrust is applied.

- The foot of the leg to be thrusted should rest just over the table end to make it more accessible to the therapist.

- Make sure to stand with one leg back to provide a stable base of support and control when applying the thrust.

- The ankle may be sensitive to grip, or its circumference too large for the therapist to effectively grip. Using a towel in place of the hands is acceptable to apply the thrust.

- Be careful not to grip too low otherwise the thrust will gap the ankle joint instead.

- Leaning back while holding the patient's leg will allow the therapist to take up the slack and will help to engage the barrier better.

- It is the abrupt contact of the elbows into the therapist's chest that limits the excursion and hence the amplitude.

- Only pull hard enough to get minimal to no movement in the head. It is speed not force that guarantees success with this technique.

- Caution should be used with this technique if the patient has a knee joint issue.

Purpose: This is a recoil technique that, according to Dr. Laurie Hartman, is one that can be used to treat a variety of SI joint dysfunctions. It is not a typical thrust technique but requires a lot of speed for performing it, especially on the release. The aim is to produce a flexion moment to the sacrum. The patient is placed in prone on the table. The therapist places their hands on either end of the sacrum. Pressure is applied through the hands to both ends of the sacrum producing somewhat of a flexion moment. Then, the hands are rapidly released from the sacrum after taking up any available slack.

When to use: Perhaps the first choice for treating SI joint dysfunctions.

Primary muscles activated: Both pectorals and minor shoulder adductors, followed by the shoulder abductors at recoil or release.

Suggested tests prior to thrust:
- Fortin's finger test.
- Sacral compression test.
- ASIS distraction test.
- Gaenslen's test.
- FABER's/Patrick's test.
- Thigh thrust/Femoral shear test.

Patient position (Figure 7.9.6a):
- Patient is prone on table.

- Can use pillow under abdomen if there is too much lumbar lordosis.

Therapist position (Figure 7.9.6a):
- Standing at side of table at the patient's pelvis.

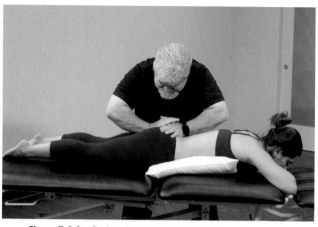

Figure 7.9.6a: Patient is prone on table and may have a pillow under the abdomen if there is too much lumbar lordosis.

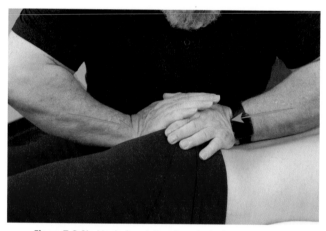

Figure 7.9.6b: Heel of each hand contacts the sacral base and sacrococcygeal region.

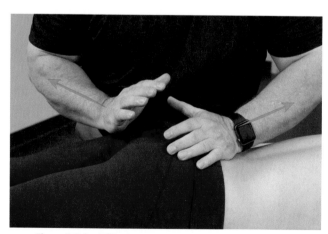

Figure 7.9.6c: With strong pressure to engage the sacrum, a very rapid release of the hands produces the recoil. This is often repeated two to three times.

Contact points (Figure 7.9.6b)**:**
- Heel of each hand will contact the sacral base and sacrococcygeal region.

Position for thrust:
- Pressure from hands is applied at about a 20-25-degree angle to the body to take up slack.

Application of technique (Figure 7.9.6b and c)**:**
- Once pressure is added to engage the sacrum, a very rapid release of the hands produces the recoil. Repeat two to three times.

Fine-tuning and keys to success:
- The table should be at a height such that the buttocks of the prone patient is at the level just below the therapist's waist.

- Therapist should flex elbows and bend to a level where the maximum amount of leverage can be used to direct pressure onto the contact areas.

- The therapist can stand with one leg back if they want to improve their control.

- The therapist's hands should be overlapped so that they are allowed to be placed accurately over the sacral base and sacrococcygeal region.

- The contact with each hand has to be very firm. A strong contraction of the pectorals is required to do this and is a preamble to successful recoil.

- Avoid intertwining the fingers as this may impede hand movement when trying to get the effect of a proper release (recoil).

- Speed of release is absolutely necessary if the therapist is going to perform this technique successfully.

- Proper alignment of the arms into the sacrum is essential to direct the force and release appropriately.

7.9.7: Pubic Thrust Technique

Purpose: This is a supine technique that is said to 'reset the pubic bones' by having the patient contract into the therapist's hands and then push the knees apart. The patient is placed in supine with their knees bent and their feet flat on the table. The therapist places their hands on the lateral aspect of both knees to resist active hip abduction. This is repeated three times with the patient starting from a more abducted position after each repetition. After this, the therapist switches their hands to the medial aspect of both knees and applies a small impulse into hip abduction while asking the patient to adduct their knees. Often you will get an articulation without applying a thrust. Many therapists will use this treatment as a preamble to treating SI joint dysfunctions.

When to use: It is used to treat pubic joint dysfunctions but is almost always done as part of treating the SI joint.

Primary muscles activated: Pectoral muscles with resistive abduction. Pectorals again with crossed arm applying the thrust into abduction.

Suggested tests prior to thrust:
- Palpation of pain and position over the symphysis pubis.

Patient position (Figure 7.9.7a and c):
- Supine with head on a pillow.

- The knees and hips are bent so that the feet rest flat on the table.

Therapist position (Figure 7.9.7a and c):
- Standing at the table next to the patient's pelvis.

Contact points:
- Initially to the outside of the patient's knees then to the inside of the patient's knees prior to the thrust.

Position for the thrust:
- Patient has flexed knees together.

- The therapist asks the patient to open the legs against resistance three times prior to repositioning the hands to the inside of the knees.

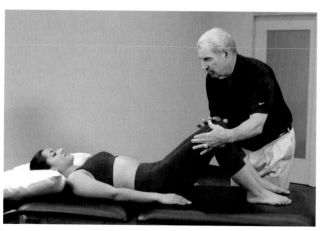

Figure 7.9.7a: Patient supine with hips and knees bent, and therapist standing at the table across from the patient's pelvis.

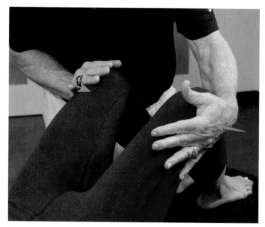

Figure 7.9.7b: Therapist provides a series of resisted hip abductions through their hands on the outside of the patient's knees.

Application of the thrust (Figure 7.9.7b and d):

- Placing the therapist's hands on the inside of each knee after the series of abductions against resistance from the outside of the patient's knees, a quick but very short amplitude thrust is performed into abduction.

Fine-tuning and keys to success:

- The table is set at a height so that the top of the patient's flexed knees are just below the level of the therapist's mid-chest. This places the therapist is the best position biomechanically to apply the thrust.

- Make sure that the application of the hands is through a wide grip so as to diffuse the force (wide contact area) on the knees.

- The contract-relax technique should be done three times and allow the legs to be abducted wider each time with the resisted abduction. The knees should be far enough apart to insert the length of the therapist's forearm between them.

- It is possible to achieve an articulation without thrusting by virtue of a contraction, but if not, apply a very short amplitude impulse into abduction to accomplish the same end.

- Crossing the arms into adduction to make contact with the inside of the patient's knees is recommended for the thrust. This allows the therapist to use their large pectoral muscles efficiently to apply the force under control.

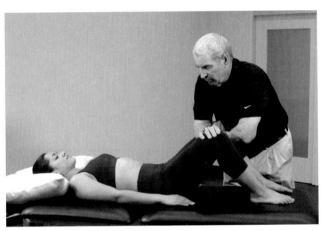

Figure 7.9.7c: Therapist switches hands to inside the patient's knees.

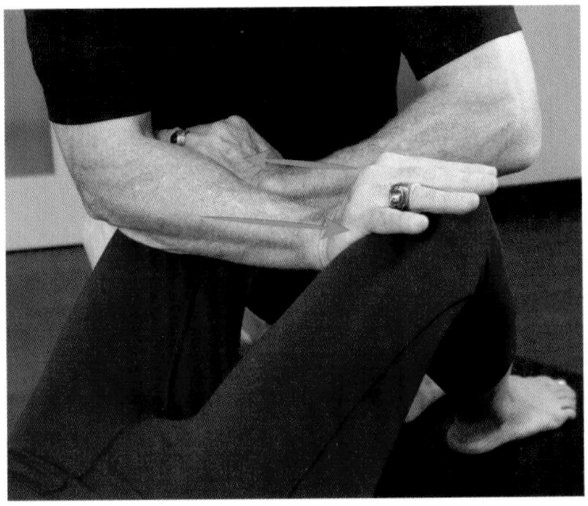

Figure 7.9.7d: Thrust is a rapid but very short amplitude movement into bilateral hip abduction while patient provides hip adduction force.

Chapter 7 References

1. Mintken PE, Derosa C, Little T, Smith B. Moving past sleight of hand. *J Orthop Sports Phys Ther*. 2010;40(5):253-255.
2. Mintken PE, DeRosa C, Little T, Smith B, American Academy of Orthopaedic Manual Physical T. AAOMPT clinical guidelines: A model for standardizing manipulation terminology in physical therapy practice. *J Orthop Sports Phys Ther*. 2008;38(3):A1-6.
3. Easton G, Stratford-Martin J, Atherton H. An appraisal of the literature on teaching physical examination skills. *Educ Prim Care*. 2012;23(4): 246-254.
4. Stagno V, Cappabianca P. See one. Do one. Teach one. A perfect paradigm for education and training in neuroendoscopy. *World Neurosurg*. 2013;79(2):258-259.
5. Kotsis SV, Chung KC. Application of the "see one, do one, teach one" concept in surgical training. *Plast Reconstr Surg*. 2013;131(5):1194-1201.
6. Johnston S. See one, do one, teach one: developing professionalism across the generations. *Clin Orthop Relat Res*. 2006;449:186-192.
7. Lenchus JD. End of the "see one, do one, teach one" era: the next generation of invasive bedside procedural instruction. *J Am Osteopath Assoc*. 2010;110(6):340-346.
8. Rodriguez-Paz JM, Kennedy M, Salas E, et al. Beyond "see one, do one, teach one": toward a different training paradigm. *Qual Saf Health Care*. 2009;18(1):63-68.
9. George JH, Doto FX. A simple five-step method for teaching clinical skills. *Fam Med*. 2001;33(8):577-578.
10. Walker MJ, Peyton JWR. Teaching in the theatre. In: Peyton JWR, ed. *Teaching and Learning in Medical Practice*: Rickmansworth: Manticone Publishing House Europe; 1998:171-180.
11. Heni M, Lammerding-Koppel M, Celebi N, et al. Focused didactic training for skills lab student tutors - which techniques are considered helpful? *GMS Z Med Ausbild*. 2012;29(3):Doc41.
12. Rossettini G, Rondoni A, Palese A, et al. Effective teaching of manual skills to physiotherapy students: a randomised clinical trial. *Med Educ*. 2017;51(8):826-838.

Chapter 8

Summary and Thoughts for the Future

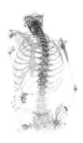

8.1: Chapter Objectives

As we stated in the preface to this book, we wanted to share our knowledge and experience primarily within our own profession, physical therapy. We are, and will always be, staunch advocates for thrust joint manipulation to remain within our professional scope of practice. However, we believe that best care of the patient should be the focal point for all providers of thrust joint manipulation. It should not matter which profession is associated with the provision of the technique as long as the patient achieves the best outcome. Unfortunately, it often seems as though we are alone in this thinking as turf wars spring up and different professions attempt to lay claim to exclusive use of thrust joint manipulation. In this final chapter, we offer a summary and some thoughts on the future direction of thrust joint manipulation as it relates to research, education, legislation and utilization.

8.2: Research Into Thrust Joint Manipulation

There is a wealth of research into the proposed mechanisms, effectiveness, comparative effectiveness, and safety of thrust joint manipulation. It is relatively easy to find randomized controlled trials and systematic reviews on the subject. Unfortunately, as we have pointed out, many of the research trials have used heterogeneous samples of subjects with spinal pain when clinical evidence strongly supports the fact that only *some* patients with spinal pain will benefit from thrust joint manipulation. Applying thrust joint manipulation to all patients with spinal pain when it is clearly perceived to be of benefit to only some patients will inevitably lead to the research findings that indicate it has no or only modest benefit. Another common problem with the research trials is that they fail to truly provide thrust joint manipulation as the intervention of interest. Studying the benefits of 'spinal manipulative therapy' for 'low back pain' inevitably becomes a study on any and all patients with low back pain who have no specific contraindications to thrust joint manipulation. And to make matters worse, 'spinal manipulative therapy' does not always include thrust joint manipulation, and instead includes non-thrust mobilizations or other forms of manual therapy.

Systematic reviews are only as good as the clinical trials that are included within the review. GIGO (Garbage In, Garbage Out) is a well-known acronym in computer science that implies bad input will result in bad output. We believe it also applies in research, and when the quality of studies is questionable at best, results of systematic reviews should be seen with a healthy dose of skepticism.

Unfortunately, because of the large numbers of studies and reviews indicating thrust joint manipulation has only poor to moderate evidence for its effectiveness over other interventions, there have been calls to stop further research on that score. There are now calls to research its cost effectiveness compared to other interventions instead. We believe that there is room for more higher quality, tightly controlled research into the effectiveness of thrust joint manipulation. Selecting appropriate subject samples and making sure thrust joint manipulation is consistently provided as the intervention should result in stronger evidence for effectiveness.

8.3: Education in Thrust Joint Manipulation

There is no doubt that education in thrust joint manipulation is extremely variable across all professions. The Commission on Accreditation in Physical Therapy Education (CAPTE) is the accrediting agency that is nationally recognized by the US Department of Education and the Council of Higher Education Accreditation. It grants specialized accreditation status to qualified entry-level education programs for physical therapists. As of April 2017, some 236 programs are accredited and they have 331,380 students enrolled in 2016-17.[1] Their published standards for accredited physical therapy education programs include Standard 7 which states that the curriculum must "include content, learning experiences, and student testing and evaluation processes designed to prepare students to achieve educational outcomes required for initial practice in physical therapy and for lifelong learning necessary for functioning within an ever-changing health care environment." The elements include 7D27(f) that requires students competently perform "manual therapy techniques (including mobilization/manipulation thrust and non-thrust techniques)."[2] As noted in chapter three, recent surveys of entry-level physical therapy program suggest that this CAPTE standard is being met, but one must question how and to what extent it is being met. Are students in all programs getting enough practical experience in thrust joint manipulation to all areas of the spine? Are students getting to put those entry-level skills into clinical practice when they are in their long-term clinical affiliations? These questions are difficult to answer.

The Council on Chiropractic Education (CCE) is the national accrediting Agency for Doctor of Chiropractic Programs within the United States.[3] As of April 2017, there were 15 programs accredited but no specific numbers of students enrolled in 2016-17 were available. Their published standards for accreditation of chiropractic programs leave no doubt that spinal adjustment/manipulation is the main focus of the education of the chiropractor. It is difficult to imagine that students in the programs are not getting enough practical experience in thrust joint manipulation to all areas of the spine, whether at school or on clinical rotations.

Osteopathy programs present an interesting dilemma because, here in the US, they are medical programs with graduates becoming medical doctors. In the US, Doctors of Osteopathy (DOs) are similar in many respects to Doctors of Medicine, and progress through residencies and specialties to work in all areas of medicine, including orthopedic surgery, internal medicine, dermatology, neurology, etc. The Commission on Osteopathic College Accreditation (COCA) is the national accrediting agency for Doctor of Osteopathy Programs in the US.[4] As of 2016, there are 33 osteopathic medical schools and they have some 27,512 students enrolled in 2016-17.[5] As part of their education, DOs receive training in the thrust joint manipulation. However, it is difficult to determine if and how many DOs actually utilize their thrust joint manipulation skills once they have graduated and entered the medical field. It is reported that 56 percent of active DOs practice in primary care specialties (family medicine, internal medicine, pediatrics, and osteopathic manipulative medicine) while the remaining 44 percent practice in all other medical specialties, with emergency medicine, general surgery, obstetrics and gynecology, anesthesiology and psychiatry being the top five.[6]

Interestingly, osteopathy programs in countries other than the US appear to be less associated with allopathic medicine and more aligned with manipulative therapy. To avoid some of this confusion, some use the term osteopathic medicine (medical) to refer to medical physicians with an osteopathic training, and osteopathy (non-medical) to refer to non-physician osteopaths who work primarily as manual or manipulative therapists. Osteopathic programs in the UK, Australia, Canada and Europe award bachelor's or master's degrees in Osteopathy.

From what has been discussed thus far, it might be tempting to suggest that, of all the professions that may practice thrust joint manipulation, physical therapy may have the least training in it. However, that would be very disingenuous. Just as clinicians from other professions may decide their career will take them into areas other than musculoskeletal medicine (and they may practice less and less thrust joint manipulation), there are many physical therapists that decide this area of clinical practice is their bailiwick. Any clinician who develops an interest and passion for thrust joint manipulation will necessarily seek ever more training and learning opportunities. It is no different for any professional.

8.4: Legislation and Thrust Joint Manipulation

There have been many attempts by the chiropractic profession to control or limit who can provide thrust joint manipulation. Opposition to physical therapists performing thrust joint manipulation started as early as the 1960s, and intensified in the 1990s in response to the physical therapy profession movement toward direct patient access and the doctoral education. As many as 23 states had legislative challenges in 1998 by the chiropractic profession. The number of legislative challenges may be less per year (typically four – eight states) but the intensity of the legislative and regulatory challenges continues even today.

Some have suggested that there was a national chiropractic agenda to own manipulation and eliminate the competition. It certainly seemed that way. In 2003, there were state legislative efforts in Hawaii, Iowa, Louisiana, New Mexico, North Dakota, Texas, and Tennessee by the chiropractic profession to prohibit manipulation performed by physical therapists based on a strategy of inadequate education. For example, they suggested a minimum of

400 hours of classroom instruction and a minimum of 800 hours of supervised clinical training in manipulation. When these efforts failed, their next strategy in 2004 was flat-out prohibition of manipulation by physical therapists in Iowa, New York, New Jersey, Oklahoma and South Carolina. For example, in South Carolina they introduced House Bill 4676 and Senate Bill 1035 which proposed that "only a licensed chiropractor may perform a specific spinal adjustment/manipulation on a patient." They defined 'adjustment or manipulation' as "the forceful movement of joints or tissue to restore joint function, in whole or part, to increase circulation, to increase motion, or to reduce\ interosseous disrelation (sic)."

During these manipulation legislative debates and negotiations, chiropractic organizations frequently express the attitude of ownership, and "manipulation is ours" seems to be their message. The physical therapy profession, of course, responds by stating (correctly) that manipulation has been a part of our practice since the birth of the profession and they provide references to prove it. The ensuing discussion then becomes nothing but a merry-go-round with nobody willing to get off the ride. The argument from the chiropractic profession is often presented as patient safety concerns, but this appears to be a smoke-screen for the real issue at hand; economics. The Institute for Alternative Futures released a document titled *The Future of Chiropractic Revisited: 2005 – 2015*.[7] In a report on the future of chiropractic, it was remarkable to find that physical therapists were mentioned on 26 different pages of the report, and well over 90 percent of the notations mentioned them in the context of an economic competitor. As an example, page vii states, "Chiropractors will face more competition, especially from the growing number of physical therapists who are pursuing direct access in all 50 states and are upgrading their educational programs to graduate Doctors of Physical Therapy." Page 13 states, "Probably the most serious competitive threat on the horizon is

from physical therapists. PT's training in and capacity to do mobilization puts them in a position to treat many of the back problems seen by chiropractors." Nowhere in the document is it mentioned that chiropractors must take action to protect the patient.

It is our contention that no single profession owns or should own this intervention that has been utilized for centuries (see Chapter 1). We believe that it should be up to the ever-more-educated consumer of these healthcare services to decide from whom they wish to receive thrust joint manipulation. If physical therapists can provide it safely and skillfully in the management of their patients with spinal pain and dysfunction, then who is to say they should not. Equally, if it is a chiropractor that provides pain relief and rehabilitation through the same thrust joint manipulation techniques, we should laud their efforts. Ultimately, we should all want what is best for the patient.

8.5: Utilization of Thrust Joint Manipulation

There is no doubt that a significant percentage of physical therapists or physiotherapists around the world do not utilize thrust joint manipulation in their daily practice. This is not a bad thing. The vision statement for the physical therapy profession is to transform society by optimizing movement to improve the human experience.[8] Optimizing movement can be achieved through many means available to the physical therapist, and it may or may not include the use of thrust joint manipulation. However, if some physical therapists discover they have a passion for and can develop significant skills in thrust joint manipulation techniques, then they should be free to do what is in the best interests of the patients they serve.

It can be argued that a significant percentage, or perhaps even the majority of chiropractors around the world *do* utilize thrust joint manipulation in their daily practice. This is also not a bad thing. However, if some chiropractors discover they do not have a great passion for, and cannot develop their skills in thrust joint manipulation techniques, then they should be just as free to provide other interventions (like exercise prescription and physical modalities) they deem appropriate for their patients.

On a final note, it is interesting that the American Chiropractic Association's vision statement includes the words "Improved health care access and freedom of choice of health care providers for the American people, without discriminatory obstacles."[9] We couldn't agree more!

8.6: Final Thoughts and Wishful Thinking About the Future

Our goal in writing this book was to provide a user-friendly resource for clinicians and student-clinicians wishing to learn how to enhance their thrust joint manipulation skills. We hope we have achieved that goal. In the process, we hope we have also contributed a little to the knowledge base on the history of manipulation, the scientific evidence for its effectiveness, the relative risks and benefits from the point of view of patient safety, and the clinically reasoned approach to its appropriate utilization.

With our combined clinical and research experience, we remain committed to the continued research of thrust joint manipulation. You could say we have 'several irons in the fire.' We are currently in the data collection stage for the validation study for the clinical prediction rule for cervical thrust joint manipulation for patients with neck pain.

We have also completed research on the intrarater reliability of the Friedman-Johnson (thoracic) tap test and hope to publish results in the near future. We also have several projects underway, including investigating the effects of neck pain on gait characteristics and the immediate effects of cervical thrust joint manipulation on those gait characteristics; the effects of neck pain on joint repositioning error and the immediate effects of thrust joint manipulation on the error rate; the localization of cavitation during thrust joint manipulation; and the effects of patient expectation on their perceptions of thrust joint manipulation to their spine. Yes, it's a lot! But we know there are just as many other researchers out there working diligently to learn as much as we can about this intervention that has been around since the time of man.

Chapter 8 References

1. APTA. Welcome to CAPTE. 2017; http://www.capteonline.org/home.aspx. Accessed 4/15/2017.
2. APTA. CAPTE Accreditation Handbook. 2017; http://www.capteonline.org/uploadedFiles/CAPTEorg/Portal/CAPTEPortal_PTStandardsEvidence.doc. Accessed 4/15/2017.
3. CCE. The Council on Chiropractic Education. 2017; http://www.cce-usa.org/Home.html. Accessed 4/15/2017.
4. AOA. American Osteopathic Association Commission on Osteopathic College Accreditation. 2017; http://www.osteopathic.org/inside-aoa/accreditation/COM-accreditation/Pages/default.aspx. Accessed 4/15/2017.
5. AOA. Osteopathic Medical Profession Report. 2017; http://www.osteopathic.org/inside-aoa/about/aoa-annual-statistics/Pages/default.aspx. Accessed 4/15/2017.
6. AOA. 2016 Osteopathic Medical Profession Report. 2017; http://www.osteopathic.org/inside-aoa/about/aoa-annual-statistics/Documents/2016-OMP-report.pdf. Accessed 4/15/2017.
7. Futures IfA. *The Future of Chiropractic Revisited*: 2005 to 2015. ww.altfutures.com2005.
8. APTA. Vision statement for the physical therapy profession. 2017; http://www.apta.org/Vision/. Accessed 4/15/2017.
9. ACA. American Chiropractic Association Vision Statement. 2017; https://www.acatoday.org/About/Mission-Vision. Accessed 4/15/2017.

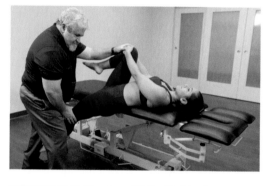

MS30500 5-Section Hi/Lo Table & RehabPro Inc.

The Hi/Lo Manual Therapy Table as seen in this book is distributed by RehabPro Inc. The armrests on this 5-Section Treatment Table are attached directly to the frame, which allows for greater vertical adjustment and easy access for cervical manipulations. The armrests can also swing out and back to increase the width of the table, allowing the extremities to rest while treating shoulders for range of motion.

RehabPro. **rehabpropulleys.com**, Therapeutic Exercise Equipment and Hi/Lo 3-Section, BoBath and Traction Tables.